Foraged & Fetched: The Evolutionary Eater's Guide

Roots & Bytes: Reclaiming Our Dietary Heritage With Modern Technology

Trevor Taylor

Roots & Bytes: Reclaiming Our Dietary Heritage With Modern Technology

indirect, that are incurred as a result of the use of the information contained within this document, including, but not limited to, errors, omissions, or inaccuracies.

Table of Contents

Foreword

As we navigate the annals of human history, the intertwined paths of biological evolution and technological advancement present a fascinating narrative of progress and imbalance. This book delves into the complex dance between our evolutionary adaptations and innovations, illustrating how shifts in this delicate balance have profound implications for our health and environment.

Our journey begins in the primitive landscapes of our ancestors, where humans' biological evolution was closely tied to the natural world. Early humans faced many challenges, from inedible and often toxic foods to harsh environmental conditions. Evolutionary traits developed over millennia, enabling us to detect and avoid natural toxins in wild plants and animals. Yet, as our societies evolved, so did our tools and techniques, gradually shifting this balance.

The discovery of fire and the development of cooking were among the first technological breakthroughs that allowed early humans to neutralize toxins in food, making previously inedible resources nutritious and safe. This leap in food processing not only expanded our dietary options but also had a profound impact on our physiological and social structures. Cooking increases nutrient absorption and caloric intake, fuels brain growth, and fosters complex social interactions.

However, the scale of advancements accelerated dramatically with the onset of agriculture and, later, the Industrial Revolution. With the advent of agriculture, humans were no longer bound by the whims of fortune inherent in hunting and gathering practices (Gunagi et al., 2019). Our ancestors could cultivate and bend the land to their will and needs. The advancements in agriculture birthed civilizations, forged empires, and propelled humanity forward on a rather relentless march of progress toward the Industrial Revolution. The advent of machines and factories set an unprecedented pace of innovation that reshaped the framework of human existence into one of efficiency and profit. These transformations allowed for control over our food sources, leading to significant societal advancements but also initiating a trend toward monocultures, processed foods, and a move away from the diverse diets of our ancestors. Contemporary agricultural practices, driven by profit and efficiency, have prioritized scale over sustainability, often at the expense of health and environmental integrity.

Today, advancements in food production have outpaced our biological needs, creating a mismatch that contributes to the global burden of chronic diseases and environmental degradation. The proliferation of processed foods, high in calories but low in nutrients, has disconnected us from the natural dietary rhythms that once governed our survival and well-being. For instance, the ubiquitous presence of fast-food establishments has become a beacon of convenience. These establishments churn out meals engineered for maximum appeal and addictive potential, laden with salt, sugar, and fat in precisely calibrated ratios designed to hijack our taste buds and override our body's satiety signals. Agribusiness conglomerates have also ushered in an era of industrialized farming practices prioritizing yield and shelf-life over nutritional quality. Genetically modified crops doused in a cocktail of pesticides and herbicides may appear appealing on supermarket shelves but are often devoid of the essential vitamins, minerals, and phytonutrients our bodies crave for optimal health.

In this brave new world of abundance, we find ourselves trapped in a paradox of plenty. Despite the abundance of calories at our fingertips, we are malnourished at a cellular level and starved for the vital nutrients that fuel our bodies and minds. Our dietary rhythms, once attuned to the ebb and flow of the seasons, now lie in disarray, disrupted by the relentless march of progress.

The consequences of this dietary discordance reverberate through every facet of our existence. Chronic diseases such as obesity, diabetes, and heart disease have reached epidemic proportions, exacting a heavy toll on both individual health and societal well-being (*Methadone for Opioid Addiction: Benefits and Risks - Haven Detox Little Rock*, 2023). Meanwhile, the environmental footprint of our modern food system looms large on the horizon, with deforestation, soil degradation, and water pollution casting a shadow over the future of our planet.

This book proposes a reawakening to the ancient wisdom that once informed human diets, combined with a critical examination of how we can use modern technology to realign our eating habits with our biological heritage. The rise of artificial intelligence offers a new hope in this regard, providing the tools to sift through vast amounts of data, debunk myths, and rediscover lost knowledge. AI can potentially be the missing link that reconnects us with our evolutionary past, and with your understanding and support, we can confidently restore balance and live more harmoniously within our ecosystems. This is not just a vision but a tangible path toward a future where our health, environment, and understanding of our place in the world are all in harmony.

Prepare to discover the symbiotic relationship between evolution and technology through vivid examples and compelling arguments. This narrative is not just an analysis of the past; it is a roadmap for navigating the complexities of the present and future, offering practical advice on leveraging AI and other technologies to achieve a healthier, more sustainable way of living. Rest assured, these changes are manageable. With your understanding and support, we can confidently restore balance and live more harmoniously within our ecosystems. Join us on this journey to rediscover the primal joy of consuming food as alive and dynamic as the world around us and learn how to harness technology to forge a future that honors our evolutionary heritage and promises a healthier and more sustainable world for all.

INTRODUCTION: OUR MODERN DISCONNECTION FROM NATURAL FOOD SOURCES

In our current era, we navigate a vast digital landscape teeming with boundless information, much like our ancestors did when exploring ancient geographical frontiers. The spirit of exploration and the allure of fulfilling our curiosity of the unknown has propelled such adventurers forward, even when the path forward becomes a dangerous labyrinth. Digital misinformation continuously proliferates, propagated by marketers, dubious influencers, and opportunistic ebook writers or bloggers. Navigating online health and nutrition information has become problematic, marked by profit-driven scams and harmful health advice.

Technological Evolution And Human Adaptation

Technological evolution has long been intertwined with human adaptation, shaping our development and survival. Current advancements in Artificial Intelligence (AI) represent a modern equivalent to historical innovations such as the creation of fire and the advent of food processing, pivotal tools driving changes in human behavior and health. These advancements, while not without their challenges, have also brought about significant improvements in our lives, such as increased food production and improved healthcare.

Early human diets were symbiotically connected to their environment, with adaptations driven by regional and seasonal availability profoundly influencing human evolution, particularly cognitive and physical developments. However, as humanity transitioned from being part of an ecological system to dominating it, the balance shifted, leading to reduced dietary diversity and increased ecological disruption, particularly with the onset of agriculture and industrialization.

Throughout history, advances in food and technology have shaped human civilization. The discovery of fire revolutionized human diet and culture, enhancing nutrient bioavailability and supporting brain development nearly a million years ago. The agricultural revolution, marked by the cultivation of crops and domestication of animals around 10,000 BCE, allowed for sedentary communities and the rise of civilizations but also introduced trends of monoculture and genetic narrowing. The mechanization of food production in the 19th century further transformed the scale and scope of food availability, increasing efficiency and giving rise to processed foods linked to health issues.

Exploring pivotal moments in food history offers invaluable insights into the delicate balance between cultural heritage and dietary risks. In Japan, for instance, the meticulous preparation of pufferfish illustrates the fine line between culinary tradition and potential lethality. This culinary artistry showcases the precision and expertise required to safely prepare and consume food that harbors deadly toxins, underscoring the complex interplay between cultural practices and dietary safety.

Similarly, the Renaissance period witnessed a dramatic expansion of global food exchanges as New World crops such as potatoes, tomatoes, and chili peppers made their way to Europe. This influx of novel foods enriched and diversified human diets and introduced new culinary possibilities. However, it also brought the inherent risks of introducing unfamiliar foods into established dietary patterns, highlighting the dynamic nature of food culture and the ever-present need for caution in embracing culinary novelties.

Tracing the evolution of food and technology throughout history reveals a deeper understanding of the intricacies that have shaped human diets and cultures. From primitive traditions to modern innovations, the story of food is a testament to humanity's ingenuity, adaptability, and resilience in the face of ever-changing culinary landscapes. How consumers understand and navigate these ever-changing culinary landscapes has also evolved.

Examining Modern Information Overload

Roetzel's review on information overload comprehensively examines consumers' present-day dilemma when inundated with a barrage of advertising and media stimuli (Roetzel, 2018). This relentless onslaught burdens individuals with decision fatigue and complicates inquiries for reliable nutritional guidance in an era where misinformation often masquerades as data-driven truth.

At the heart of Roetzel's insights is the recognition that today's consumer is bombarded with unprecedented information, much of which is tailored to capture attention rather than convey accurate nutritional advice. In this landscape, marketing and advertising campaigns often prioritize engagement metrics over factual accuracy, leading to misleading claims and half-truths.

As a result, consumers find themselves lost in a web of fad diets, miracle supplements, and dubious health claims. The result is pervasive confusion and uncertainty as individuals need help to discern credible information from cleverly crafted marketing ploys. Moreover, the rise of influencer culture has further complicated matters, as individuals with little to no expertise in nutrition or health are elevated to positions of authority based solely on their social media following. The result is a proliferation of unqualified voices peddling advice, further muddying the waters for consumers seeking trustworthy guidance.

Critical thinking and media literacy have never been more urgent in this climate. Roetzel's review underscores the importance of empowering consumers to question the information sources they encounter and seek evidence-based resources backed by scientific rigor. By arming themselves with the tools necessary to navigate the digital landscape, individuals can better protect themselves from misinformation and make informed decisions about their health and well-being.

Ai's Role In Cutting Through Misinformation

In this information age, artificial intelligence emerges as a beacon of hope, promising to cut through the information noise to provide clarity and precision. Integrating artificial intelligence with nutrition science practices has ushered in a new era of data analytics and personalized nutrition. AI algorithms are revolutionizing how researchers sift through vast repositories of scientific studies, enabling them to extract valuable insights, validate hypotheses, and debunk myths with unprecedented speed and accuracy.

By leveraging machine learning techniques, AI can analyze extensive datasets from diverse sources, ranging from clinical trials to population studies, in a fraction of the time it would take traditional research methods. This allows researchers to identify patterns, correlations, and causal relationships that may have eluded detection through conventional means. For example, AI algorithms can sift through all available nutritional data to uncover associations between dietary factors and health outcomes, shedding light on the complex interplay between nutrition and disease.

Moreover, AI is harnessed to provide personalized diet recommendations tailored to individual genetic makeup, lifestyle factors, and health data. By integrating genetic information, biomarkers, and other relevant data points, AI algorithms can generate personalized nutrition plans that optimize health outcomes for each individual. For instance, AI-powered platforms can analyze genetic predispositions to specific dietary sensitivities or metabolic traits, allowing for targeted dietary interventions that maximize efficacy and minimize adverse effects.

Furthermore, AI-driven personalized nutrition platforms can consider lifestyle factors such as activity levels, sleep patterns, and stress levels, providing holistic recommendations that address the multifaceted nature of human health. By continuously analyzing and adapting to user data, these platforms can refine and optimize dietary recommendations, ensuring they remain aligned with individual health goals and preferences.

Overall, integrating AI into nutrition science holds immense promise for advancing our understanding of the complex relationship between diet and health and empowering individuals to make informed dietary choices tailored to their unique needs and circumstances. As AI technologies continue to evolve and mature, they have the potential to revolutionize the field of nutrition and usher in a new era of personalized, precision nutrition.

Conclusion: Harnessing The New Frontier

Navigating the vast trove of nutritional information inundating our world reveals that cautious innovation is paramount. AI is a powerful tool in this endeavor, enabling us to sift through the noise and reclaim a refined nourishment understanding. However, as we navigate this new frontier, it is essential to maintain a balanced approach that respects historical dietary wisdom and the precision of modern technology.

By marrying the insights of our ancestral past with the potential of AI-driven data analytics, we can address contemporary health challenges with newfound clarity and efficacy. This approach allows us to honor our evolutionary heritage's legacy while harnessing innovation's transformative power. By embracing this balanced approach, we pave the way toward a healthier and more sustainable tomorrow for future generations. By harnessing the power of AI with cautious innovation, we can navigate the complexities of our world and carve out a path toward optimal health and well-being. As we continue, let us remain steadfast in our commitment to honoring the wisdom of the past while embracing the possibilities of the future.

CHAPTER 1: ROOTS OF NOURISHMENT

Understanding Our Ancestral Diet

The relationship between humans and food has been a cornerstone of our existence. Understanding our ancestors' dietary practices provides insight into the origins of nutritional theories and sheds light on the intricate interplay between diet, health, and wellness.

Food has always been more than mere sustenance; it's been woven into the fabric of our beings, shaping our cultures, societies, and, ultimately, our health and well-being. Delving into the dietary practices of our ancestors not only illuminates the roots of modern nutritional theories but also unveils the intricate dance between diet, health, and wellness that has persisted throughout human history.

Anthropological studies serve as invaluable data points in this exploration, offering glimpses into the dietary habits of our hunter-gatherer forebears. It's been revealed that these primitive diets were predominantly plant-based, comprising approximately 65% plant foods and 35% animal-based foods. Take, for instance, the Yanomami tribe, whose diet is rich in forest foods, providing them with over 3.5 ounces of fiber daily—a staggering contrast to the fiber-deprived contemporary diets prevalent in many developed nations (Moubtahij et al., 2024).

But the story doesn't end with our ancestors. Today, there are still pockets of humanity whose dietary habits harken back to those of our hunter-gatherer predecessors. One such group is the Hadza people of Tanzania, whose lifestyle and diet offer a living testament to the health-promoting qualities of foodways. Despite living in a world increasingly dominated by processed foods and sedentary lifestyles, the Hadza maintain a diet rich in wild plant foods, game meat, and honey, mirroring the dietary diversity of their ancient ancestors.

Remarkably, the health of the Hadza stands in stark contrast to that of many Western populations. With minimal incidence of present-day diseases such as diabetes and cardiovascular issues, the Hadza offers a compelling case study of the potential health benefits of aligning our diets with the practices of our hunter-gatherer past. Their robust health and vitality are a powerful reminder of dietary choices' profound impact on human health and well-being.

The Hadza people's narrative reflects our shared human history and is a beacon of hope for the future of nutrition and health. By embracing the lessons of our ancestors and returning to a diet centered around whole, unprocessed foods, we can reclaim our birthright of vibrant health and vitality, paving the way for a brighter, healthier future for future generations.

Historical Relationship In Hunter-Gatherer Societies

The dietary practices of hunter-gatherer societies offer valuable lessons in sustainability, diversity, and adaptation. The transition from nomadic hunter-gatherer lifestyles to settled agrarian civilizations was pivotal in human history, shaping our societies, diets, and food production techniques. To understand the evolution of nutritional lifestyles, let's explore the agricultural practices of historical civilizations, focusing on ancient Rome as a case study, as well as contrasting it with the seasonal foraging practices of the San people in the Kalahari Desert and the marine hunting traditions of the Inuit in the Arctic.

Agricultural Practices of Old Civilizations

The transition from hunter-gatherer societies to agricultural civilizations marked a significant shift in dietary patterns and food production techniques. In ancient Rome, staple foods such as grains, mainly wheat and barley, formed the foundation of the diet. The Romans adapted agricultural techniques to support large urban populations, emphasizing the centrality of grain in their culinary traditions.

Ancient Rome: The Breadbasket of Civilization

Romans consumed a diet heavily reliant on grains such as farro and spelt, complemented by olives, grapes, and meats during festive occasions. Agricultural innovations such as aqueducts and irrigation systems enabled the cultivation of vast tracts of land, transforming Rome into the breadbasket of civilization.

The annual festival of Saturnalia provides a vivid snapshot of Roman dietary customs and cultural traditions. During this celebration, foods harvested throughout the year were shared among all social classes, symbolizing abundance and communal solidarity.

Seasonal Foraging: The Wisdom of the San People

In stark contrast to the agricultural practices of ancient Rome, the San people of the Kalahari Desert relied on seasonal foraging for their sustenance. Their diet consisted of various plants and animals, with mongongo nuts serving as a primary source of calories and nutrients. During certain seasons, mongongo nuts provided up to 50% of their caloric intake, highlighting the importance of seasonal variation in their diet.

The San people's deep knowledge of their environment enabled them to navigate the desert landscape precisely, exploiting the seasonal abundance of resources. Specific plants and animals, such as the nutritious mongongo nuts and game animals, played vital roles in their diet and cultural practices.

A day in the life of a San forager offers a glimpse into their intimate connection to the land and its cycles. From gathering wild fruits and tubers to hunting small game, each activity is guided by centuries of accumulated wisdom passed down through generations.

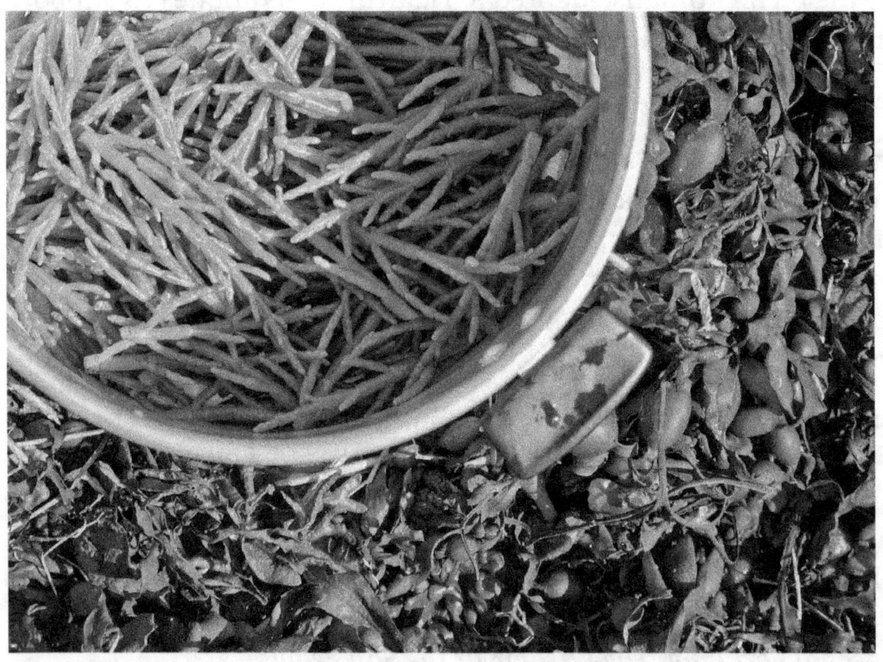

Marine Hunting: The Resilience of the Inuit

In the unforgiving terrain of the Arctic, the Inuit people relied on marine hunting for survival. Seal fat, rich in vitamin D and omega-3 fatty acids, provided essential nutrition in an environment where plant foods were scarce. Every part of the animal was utilized, reflecting the Inuit's profound respect for the ecosystem and their resourceful approach to subsistence living.

Seal hunting was central to Inuit culture and livelihoods, with techniques passed down through oral tradition and practiced with meticulous attention to detail. Seal fat, in particular, played a critical role in their diet, providing essential nutrients for health and well-being in a harsh and unforgiving environment.

Traditional Inuit hunting practices are steeped in ritual and reverence for the natural world. From the construction of *qajaq* (kayaks) to the art of harpooning seals, each hunt aspect is imbued with cultural significance and ecological wisdom.

Dietary Customs During the Renaissance
In the Renaissance era in Europe, the arrival of new foods from the Americas reshaped dietary norms, ushering in a period of culinary transformation. Dietary practices underwent a profound shift by introducing ingredients such as tomatoes and potatoes, previously unknown to European palates. This newfound abundance spurred an increase in the consumption of sugar and meats among the affluent classes, marking the beginnings of dietary excess.

However, alongside this culinary opulence emerged early signs of societal disparities in access to food. While the wealthy indulged in lavish feasts adorned with exotic delicacies, the peasantry grappled with limited access to such luxuries; their diets predominantly comprised staples like grains and vegetables.

In particular, introducing tomatoes and potatoes brought opportunities and challenges to European diets. At the same time, these novel foods enriched culinary traditions and diversified gastronomic offerings; they also posed nutritional challenges due to their unfamiliarity and potential misconceptions about their consumption.

At the heart of Renaissance society were grand feasts, where the stark differences between the diets of the wealthy and the peasantry were fully displayed. Lavish banquets hosted by nobility featured extravagant spreads of exotic meats, rare spices, and decadent desserts, showcasing the abundance enjoyed by the privileged few. In contrast, the diets of the peasantry were characterized by simplicity and frugality, with meals centered around essential ingredients sourced from local farms and gardens.

These Renaissance feasts served as microcosms of the broader societal divisions, highlighting the disparities in access to food and the unequal distribution of culinary wealth. Yet, they also symbolized the cultural richness and diversity that emerged from the mingling of different culinary traditions, shaping the gastronomic landscape of Europe for centuries to come.

Traditional Food Processing Techniques

Civilizations developed ingenious food processing techniques to enhance their diets' safety and nutritional value. Fermentation, soaking, and sprouting were employed to reduce anti-nutrients like lectins, phytates, and goitrogens, ensuring that foods were palatable and nourishing.

The Art of Fermentation

Fermentation is a natural biochemical process that has been harnessed by various cultures for centuries to preserve foods and enhance their nutritional profile. At its core, fermentation involves the conversion of carbohydrates into organic acids, gasses, or alcohol by microorganisms such as bacteria, yeast, or fungi. This transformative process extends the shelf life of foods and enhances their flavor, texture, and digestibility. One significant benefit of fermentation is the reduction of harmful compounds like lectins in grains and legumes. Lectins are anti-nutrients in many plant-based foods that can interfere with digestion and nutrient absorption.

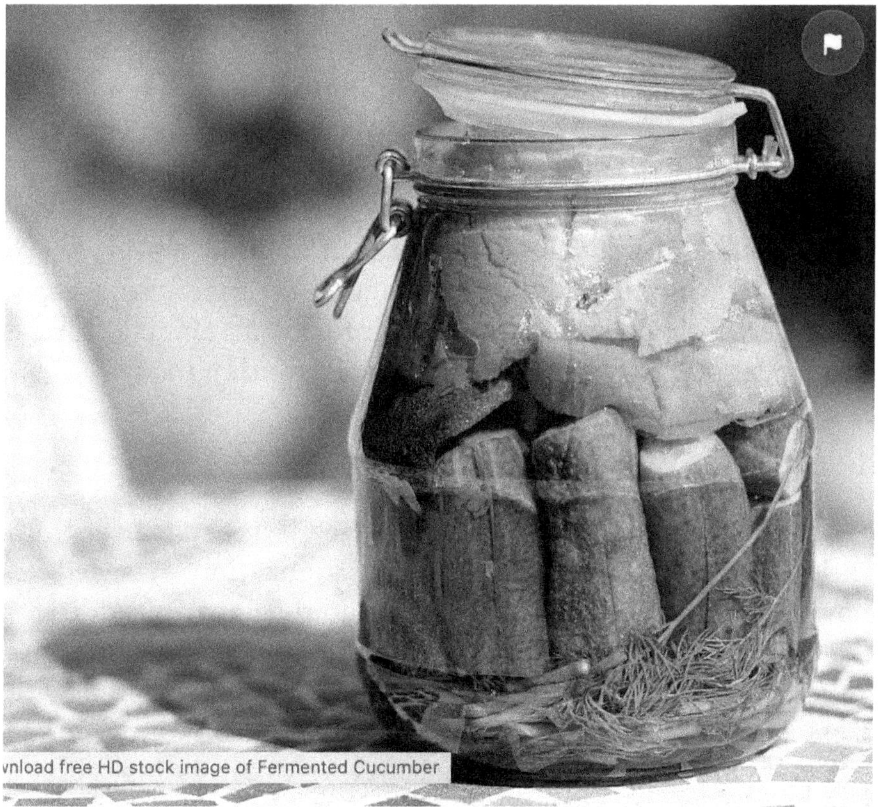

A classic example of fermentation in action is the traditional Korean practice of kimchi-making. Kimchi is a staple in Korean cuisine, a spicy and tangy fermented vegetable dish typically made with cabbage and radishes. The process of making kimchi involves community participation and highlights the cultural importance of food processing techniques in Korean society. The communal aspect of kimchi-making is central to its cultural significance. Families and communities often come together to prepare large kimchi batches, which are shared and enjoyed throughout the year. This sense of shared effort and tradition underscores the importance of food in Korean culture and highlights fermentation's role in preserving food and heritage.

Preserving Life in Ice Cellars

In the frozen landscapes where the Inuit thrive, ingenuity led to the development of ice cellars—subterranean storage spaces carved into permafrost that served as natural freezers. These ice cellars kept hunted seals, whales, and caribou fresh throughout the year, demonstrating a profound understanding of the environment and a sustainable approach to food preservation. This practice highlights how indigenous technologies, deeply rooted in ecological awareness, could inform sustainable storage solutions, reducing energy use in food preservation today.

The Shift Toward Food Processing

The advent of food processing has seen a departure from traditional beneficial practices. Industrialization has led to removing critical dietary fibers and adding harmful additives for convenience and extended shelf life, resulting in a loss of nutritional value and increased health risks associated with processed foods. The post-Industrial Revolution era marked significant changes in diet and health, closely correlating with an uptick in chronic diseases. Since the late 20th century, the rise of processed food consumption has paralleled an increase in obesity rates, diabetes, and cardiovascular diseases globally. In the U.S., obesity rates climbed from 15% in the early 1970s to over 42% by 2020. Concurrently, diabetes prevalence nearly doubled from 1980 to 2014, underscoring the health impacts of dietary shifts toward high-calorie, low-nutrient foods (Temple, 2022).

TV Dinners and Health Decline

The mid-20th-century American landscape saw a dramatic shift toward convenience foods, exemplified by the popularity of TV dinners introduced in the 1950s. These quick, ready-to-eat meals catered to the burgeoning number of dual-income households and the growing reliance on television for leisure. However, this shift also marked a decline in dietary quality, heavily incorporating high-fructose corn syrup and other additives by the 1970s. In the subsequent decades, we witnessed a stark rise in health issues like obesity and heart disease, highlighting the profound impact of processed foods on American health metrics.

Modern Dietary Missteps

Industrial farming techniques and the proliferation of processed foods have raised ethical and environmental concerns, contrasting starkly with the sustainable practices of hunter-gatherer societies. The usage of high-fructose corn syrup (HFCS) and trans fats in processed foods has been linked to rising rates of obesity, diabetes, and heart disease, highlighting the detrimental effects of present-day dietary trends

Industrial Farming and Processed Foods

Industrial farming and the widespread use of antibiotics in agriculture have profound implications for both human health and animal welfare. According to the CDC, antibiotic resistance leads to approximately 23,000 deaths annually in the United States alone, and a staggering 80% of total antibiotics used in the country are administered in agriculture (Dadgostar, 2019). This alarming statistic raises concerns about the emergence of drug-resistant bacteria, posing a significant threat to public health.

To understand the impact of industrial farming practices on antibiotic usage and resistance, let's reflect on the evolution of a poultry farm from traditional methods to intensive factory farming. Initially, traditional farming practices relied on minimal antibiotic usage, with farmers primarily administering antibiotics to treat specific illnesses or infections in their livestock. However, as the demand for poultry products grew and industrial farming methods became prevalent, the use of antibiotics escalated dramatically.

In intensive factory farming operations, where large numbers of animals are confined in close quarters, antibiotics are often administered prophylactically to prevent the outbreak of diseases that can spread rapidly in such crowded conditions. This widespread and indiscriminate use of antibiotics impacts animal welfare by masking poor living conditions and promoting the growth of antibiotic-resistant bacteria within the animals' bodies. It also contributes to the proliferation of drug-resistant pathogens in the environment.

As a result, the evolution of poultry farming practices toward intensive factory farming has led to a concerning rise in antibiotic usage, with detrimental effects on animal and human health. The overuse of antibiotics in agriculture not only compromises the efficacy of these life-saving drugs for human medical treatment but also perpetuates a cycle of antibiotic resistance that poses a significant public health threat.

High-Fructose Corn Syrup Usage

The consumption of high-fructose corn syrup rose significantly to 60 pounds per person annually by 2000, coinciding with a sharp increase in obesity rates in the United States during the same period (Klurfeld et al., 2012). A generational dietary shift from balanced diets to HFCS-laden foods has been observed, leading to adverse health effects such as obesity and diabetes.

Trans Fats and Fast Food

Following the trans fat ban in New York City, there were notable reductions in heart disease incidents, showcasing the effectiveness of nutritional policy on public health. The narrative delves into New York City's legislative efforts to ban trans fats, underscoring this landmark decision's broader public health significance.

Genetically Modified Organisms (GMOs):

Transitioning from traditional to genetically modified organism crops can significantly affect farmers, land use, pesticide dependency, and farm biodiversity. Initially, the farmer relies on traditional farming methods, cultivating heirloom or conventional crop varieties using established agricultural practices. These methods often involve crop rotation, natural fertilizers, and minimal pesticide use, fostering biodiversity and soil health.

However, farmers consider transitioning to GMO crops as the demand for higher yields and pest resistance grows. GMOs are engineered to possess desirable traits such as resistance to pests, diseases, or herbicides, promising increased productivity and reduced crop losses. The farmer may experience changes in land use patterns upon adopting GMO crops. With the introduction of pest-resistant GMOs, the need for crop rotation and diverse plantings diminishes, leading to monoculture farming practices. Large swathes of land are dedicated to growing a single GMO crop variety, potentially reducing farm biodiversity and ecosystem resilience.

Furthermore, GMO cultivation often goes hand in hand with heightened pesticide use. While GMOs engineered for pest resistance may initially reduce the need for insecticides, they often lead to increased herbicide usage. Herbicide-resistant GMO crops allow farmers to apply potent herbicides like glyphosate more liberally, resulting in the emergence of herbicide-resistant weeds and the need for more robust chemical interventions.

The widespread adoption of GMO crops raises concerns about their long-term impacts on farm biodiversity and sustainability. Monoculture farming practices associated with GMO cultivation can lead to the loss of native plant species, disruption of natural ecosystems, and decreased resilience to pests and diseases.

Nutritional And Health Benefits Of A Hunter-Gatherer Diet

Anthropological Studies and Nutritional Research

In contrast, hunter-gatherer diets are characterized by their diversity, nutrient density, and reliance on whole, unprocessed foods. Compared with today's agricultural products, hunter-gatherer diets rich in wild foods exhibit higher omega-3 and lower saturated fat levels. Research on populations such as the ! Kung San and the Kitava Islanders have shown low incidences of chronic diseases, underscoring the health benefits of traditional dietary practices. The !Kung exhibits low hypertension rates, and Kitava inhabitants show minimal cardiovascular disease, exemplifying how diet and lifestyle changes have negatively impacted our health (Lee, 1979; Lindeberg et al., 1999).

Studies on populations such as the Hadza tribe in Tanzania have revealed the importance of dietary fiber in promoting gut health and diversity, highlighting the role of diet in shaping the microbiome and overall health outcomes. Research on grains like quinoa and amaranth has demonstrated their superior nutritional profile compared to modern refined grains, further emphasizing the importance of incorporating whole, unprocessed foods into the diet.

Due to their high nutrient content, grains like quinoa and amaranth are associated with lower risks of diabetes and heart disease. There has been a renewed interest in ancient grains, driven by their exceptional nutritional profiles and perceived health benefits in recent years. These grains are rich in fiber, protein, vitamins, minerals, and antioxidants, making them valuable components of a balanced diet. Moreover, many grains are gluten-free or have lower gluten content than modern wheat, catering to individuals with gluten sensitivities or dietary restrictions.

Conclusion: The Need For A Return To Basics

In conclusion, the insights gleaned from studying ancestral diets highlight the importance of integrating lessons from our past into current eating practices. Advocating for a return to whole, unprocessed foods can help mitigate the health risks associated with contemporary dietary trends and enhance overall well-being. Furthermore, by leveraging the power of AI to analyze nutritional data and optimize food processing techniques, we can reintegrate the beneficial aspects of ancient dietary wisdom into health strategies, thereby paving the way for a healthier and more sustainable future.

Individually, we can prioritize whole, unprocessed foods, incorporate more plant-based meals into our diets, and support local and sustainable food systems. These informed choices not only promote personal health but also contribute to the well-being of the planet.

However, individual actions alone are insufficient. Policy changes are imperative to establish environments that foster healthy eating habits and sustainable food production. Governments and policymakers are pivotal in implementing regulations that facilitate access to nutritious foods, incentivize sustainable farming practices, and regulate harmful food additives and ingredients.

In the next chapter, we delve into the historical significance of hunting for survival and connection with nature. From antiquated to contemporary times, we redefine today's hunter as an individual who seeks nutritionally rich, unadulterated, and sustainably sourced foods. Driven by a profound respect for nature and our bodies, this hunter deeply understands the importance of nourishing oneself while honoring the natural world.

CHAPTER 2: THE HUNTER'S WAY

Introduction: Reviving the Hunter's Ethos

Hunting has long been embedded in human history as more than just a means of survival; it embodies a profound connection with nature. Ancient hunters navigated their environments with an intimate understanding of animal behaviors, migration patterns, and seasonal changes. Beyond securing sustenance, hunting was a sacred ritual, a dance with the natural world's rhythms, fostering a deep respect for the life it sustained. Ancient hunters were intricately attuned to their surroundings, relying on centuries of accumulated wisdom to navigate diverse terrains and ecosystems. For instance, Native American tribes like the Apache demonstrated unparalleled skill in tracking and hunting game, their techniques honed through generations of observation and adaptation. This deep connection with the land fostered a symbiotic relationship with nature, where mutual respect and stewardship were paramount.

In today's world, the essence of hunting lives on in a different guise. The present-day 'hunter' no longer wields spears and arrows but ventures into supermarkets and farmers' markets armed with nutrition, ethics, and knowledge about eco-friendliness. This contemporary form of hunting is driven by a similar ethos—a quest for nutritionally rich, unadulterated, and sustainably sourced foods that honor nature and our bodies. For example, the rise of certifications like Fair Trade and USDA Organic in supermarkets reflects this new hunting ground where consumers use labels to 'track' the origins and implications of their food choices. Just as ancient hunters tracked game through the wilderness, consumers trace the origins of their food, ensuring that each purchase aligns with their principles and beliefs.

The Hunter's Transformation: From Ancient To Contemporary

The evolution of the hunter's role parallels humanity's journey through time, from the primal necessity of survival to a present-day quest for ethical and sustainable nourishment. We have introduced how the ancient practice of hunting for sustenance has transformed into a symbolic act of selecting foods that align with health values, ethics, and environmental stewardship. Now, let us dive deeper into the evolution of human hunting practices.

Evolution of Hunting Practices

Historically, hunting was not merely a means of procuring food; it shaped social structures, cultural rituals, and even migration patterns. For instance, the Maasai tribes of Africa have long relied on the migratory patterns of the Serengeti wildebeests, aligning their hunting practices with the rhythms of wildlife for centuries. This deep connection with nature underscored a reverence for the land and its inhabitants, mirroring hunters' historical respect for their ecosystems.

Today, hunting has transcended physical tracking to become a symbolic pursuit of green sourcing and informed purchasing.

Consumers, reminiscent of primitive hunters, are now tasked with understanding the origins of their food and the broader impact of their choices on their health and the health of the environment around them. For example, opting for a locally produced apple over an imported one at a farmers' market reflects a decision informed by considerations of carbon footprints and local economic support—values deeply rooted in the ethos of ancient hunting communities.

The transition into symbolic hunting has spurred a seismic shift in market trends, with consumers driving demand for organically produced foods. This demand has catalyzed a significant expansion of organic farmland across the United States, as evidenced by a 50% increase in sales of organic foods from 2011 to 2016, according to the USDA (Skorbiansky et al., 2023). As today's hunters embrace principled sourcing practices, they have considerable influence on the future of food production and consumption.

From the hunting grounds of old civilizations to the aisles of modern supermarkets, the hunter's journey reflects humanity's ongoing quest for connection with nature and nourishment. By adopting the principles of ethical sourcing and informed decision-making, hunters honor the legacy of their ancestors while creating a healthier and more sustainable future.

The Power Of Informed Choices

In a world inundated with food options, the power of informed choices represents hope for both personal health and environmental greenness. Let us explore the profound impact of selecting sustainably sourced foods, tracing the lineage of this practice back to the selective and purposeful approach of our hunter-gatherer ancestors.

Choosing Sustainably Sourced Foods

Choosing eco-friendly sourced foods, such as local produce, free-range meats, and organic products, carries far-reaching implications for individuals and the planet. By supporting local farmers and producers, consumers ensure fresher, more nutritious fare and reduce carbon emissions associated with transportation. Furthermore, opting for free-range meats and organic products minimizes exposure to harmful chemicals and promotes animal welfare, fostering a healthier ecosystem. At the core of sustainable food choices lies a philosophy akin to that of the early hunter-gatherer: the desire to survive and thrive. Our ancestors approached food discerningly, selecting only the most nourishing and abundant sources available in their ecosystems.

The Evolution of Hunting Tools

The evolution of hunting tools offers a striking parallel to today's transition toward more humane and environmentally friendly hunting technologies. From crude stone implements to sophisticated metal weapons, the trajectory of hunting tools mirrors humanity's increasing awareness of the necessity for ethical and green practices. Modern hunters now utilize biodegradable bullets and non-toxic lead alternatives, minimizing environmental impact and promoting responsible stewardship of natural resources.

By embracing conscientious hunting practices, hunters inspire informed consumer choices among the broader population. As consumers become more aware of food source environmental footprints, they make decisions that are more aligned with health and eco-friendly practices. In this way, the power of informed choices transcends individual actions, catalyzing a collective movement toward a more resilient and harmonious relationship with our food systems and the natural world.

Community Influence And Market Trends

Every community is at the heart of interconnected choices that collectively shape individual well-being and broader societal and environmental health. An intricate relationship exists between individual and family choices, community influence, and market trends. These powerful relationships often fuel grassroots actions that catalyze transformative shifts toward more sustainable practices.

The Power of Local Choices

Individual and family choices locally wield remarkable influence over community health and well-being. Whether opting for locally sourced produce, supporting small-scale farmers, or choosing sustainable products, each decision ripples outward, contributing to the resilience and vitality of the community ecosystem. By fostering a culture of conscious consumption, communities can cultivate environments that prioritize responsible, healthy practices.

Shifting Market Trends With Community Influence

Every purchase is a potent signal to businesses, offering insights into consumer values and preferences. Individuals and families align their purchasing decisions with conscientious considerations, creating a demand for responsibly sourced and environmentally friendly products. This collective demand, aggregated across communities, can catalyze industry-wide changes, prompting businesses to reevaluate their practices and embrace more sustainable approaches to production and consumption.

Throughout history, communities have been pivotal in driving positive change through their consumption habits and advocacy efforts. From grassroots movements advocating for fair trade and organic certification to local initiatives promoting community-supported agriculture (CSA) and farmers' markets, examples abound of how communities have leveraged their collective power to influence market trends and foster greener practices. By amplifying voices at the local level, communities can affect systemic change through 'bottom-up' advocacy.

Empowering Consumer Choice

In an increasingly interconnected world, consumers have unprecedented access to information and resources that empower them to make informed purchase choices. By educating themselves about the environmental, social, and ethical implications of their consumption habits, individuals and families can become agents of change within their communities. Through conscious consumption and advocacy, they can drive demand for products that prioritize people and the planet, inspiring businesses to adopt more sustainable practices and catalyzing a global shift toward a regenerative economy.

Individuals and families make conscious choices locally, contributing to broader shifts in market dynamics and driving demand for products and practices that prioritize environmental and social responsibility. By harnessing the power of collective action and advocacy, communities can affect transformative change, creating a more equitable, resilient, and sustainable future for generations to come.

Tools For The Today's Hunter

Seasonal Food Guides

Seasonal food guides serve as invaluable resources for today's conscientious consumers. They offer insights into the natural rhythms of agricultural production and the optimal times for harvesting or purchasing local produce. Much like the early almanacs that guided traditional hunters and gatherers, today's guides provide a roadmap for aligning food choices with the ebb and flow of the seasons, fostering a deeper connection to the land and reducing reliance on out-of-season imports.

Understanding Seasonal Patterns

A deep understanding of natural cycles and environmental cues lies at the heart of seasonal food guides. By recognizing the seasonal availability of various fruits, vegetables, and other agricultural products, consumers can make more informed choices about their food purchases. This knowledge not only supports local farmers by promoting the consumption of in-season produce but also reduces the environmental footprint associated with long-distance transportation and out-of-season cultivation.

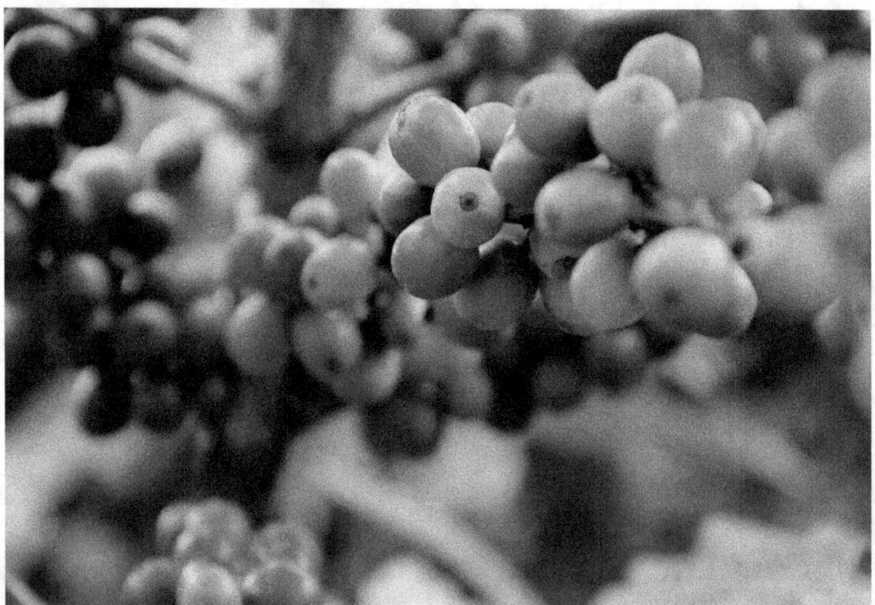

Supporting Local Agriculture

Seasonal food guides are crucial in bolstering local agriculture and strengthening community resilience. By encouraging consumers to prioritize locally grown and seasonal produce, these guides help sustain small-scale farmers and preserve agricultural diversity. Moreover, by fostering direct relationships between producers and consumers, seasonal food guides promote transparency and accountability in the food system, empowering individuals to make choices that align with their values and priorities.

Reducing Environmental Impacts

One of the most significant benefits of seasonal food guides is their potential to reduce the environmental impacts of food production and distribution. By opting for in-season, locally sourced produce, consumers can minimize the carbon emissions associated with transportation and storage and reduce the need for synthetic fertilizers and pesticides. Additionally, supporting local agriculture helps conserve water resources, protect biodiversity, and mitigate the adverse effects of industrial farming practices on soil health and ecosystem integrity.

In an era of globalized food systems and industrialized agriculture, seasonal food guides empower consumers seeking to make more sustainable and ethical food choices. By arming themselves with knowledge about seasonal patterns and local agricultural practices, individuals can become stewards of their food environment, supporting regenerative farming practices, promoting food sovereignty, and fostering resilient, community-centered food systems.

Farmers' Markets

Direct Producer-Consumer Relationships

At the heart of farmers' markets lies the principle of direct producer-consumer relationships, bypassing the intermediaries of traditional retail channels. By engaging directly with farmers, artisans, and food producers, consumers gain unparalleled insight into the origins of their food, fostering transparency and accountability in the supply chain. This direct connection allows individuals to ask questions, share stories, and forge meaningful relationships with the people who grow and harvest their food, enhancing the sense of community and trust.

Learning and Education

Farmers' markets serve as invaluable educational platforms, offering consumers opportunities to deepen their understanding of sustainable farming practices, environmental stewardship, and seasonal eating. Through workshops, cooking demonstrations, and educational events, market-goers can learn about topics ranging from organic agriculture and permaculture to food preservation and nutrition. Farmers' markets empower individuals to make informed choices that align with their values and priorities by fostering a lifelong learning and curiosity culture.

Supporting Local Economies

Beyond their role as hubs of education and community engagement, farmers' markets play a vital economic role in supporting local economies and small-scale agriculture. By providing a direct market for local farmers and artisans, these gatherings bolster rural livelihoods, preserve agricultural traditions, and contribute to the vitality of rural communities. Additionally, the economic multiplier effect of dollars spent at farmers' markets reverberates throughout the local economy, generating employment opportunities and stimulating growth in related sectors.

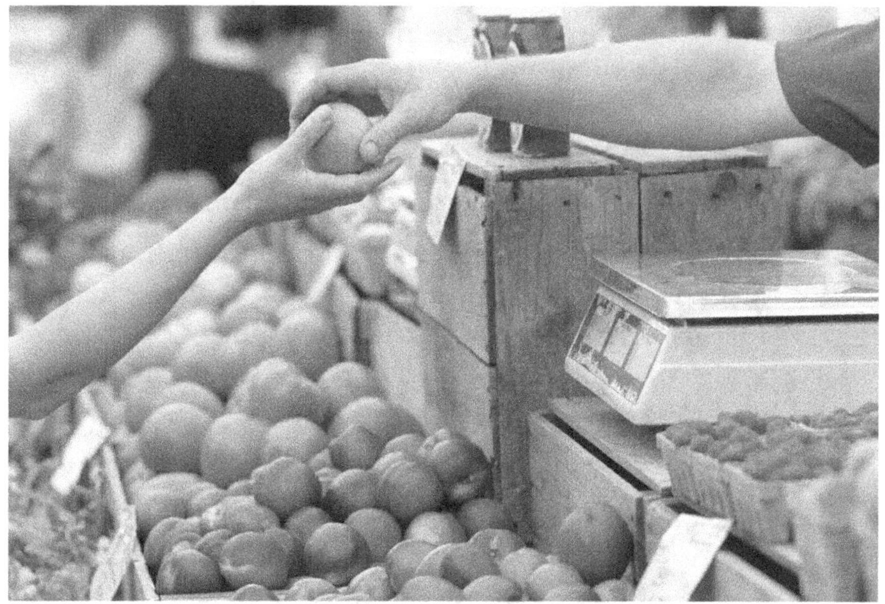

Promoting Environmental Sustainability

In an era marked by concerns about climate change, biodiversity loss, and food insecurity, farmers' markets emerge as beacons of environmental sustainability. Promoting local and seasonal eating, reducing food miles, and minimizing packaging waste, these gatherings help mitigate the environmental impacts of food production and distribution. Moreover, by supporting regenerative agricultural practices such as organic farming, agroforestry, and permaculture, farmers' markets contribute to soil health, water conservation, and ecosystem resilience.

Certifications and Labels

Certifications and labels are visual indicators of a product's adherence to specific standards, criteria, or values set forth by certifying organizations. These designations are displayed prominently on product packaging and provide consumers with tangible evidence of a product's attributes, such as organic farming practices, fair labor standards, or environmental sustainability. By evaluating and comparing these labels, consumers can navigate the complexities of the food marketplace and make choices that reflect their personal beliefs and preferences.

Examples of Certifications and Labels:

1. **Organic Certification:** The USDA Organic label is one of the most well-known certifications. It indicates that a product has been produced using organic farming methods free from synthetic pesticides, fertilizers, and genetically modified organisms. This label assures consumers that the product meets stringent standards for environmental stewardship, animal welfare, and biodiversity conservation.

2. **Rainforest Alliance:** The Rainforest Alliance Certified seal signifies that a product has been sourced from farms or forests that meet rigorous criteria, including protecting wildlife habitat, conserving natural resources, and promoting the rights and well-being of farm workers and local communities. Products bearing this label support responsible land management practices and contribute to preserving vital ecosystems.

3. **Fair Trade Certification:** The Fair Trade Certified label indicates that a product has been sourced from producers who adhere to fair labor practices. This ensures farmers receive fair crop prices, engage in equitable trade relationships, and invest in community development projects. This label empowers consumers to support ethical supply chains and promote social justice in the global marketplace.

4. **Non-GMO Project Verified:** The Non-GMO Project Verified seal assures consumers that a product does not contain genetically modified organisms or genetically engineered ingredients. This label provides

transparency and peace of mind for individuals seeking to avoid GMOs and supports agricultural practices prioritizing environmental friendliness and consumer health.

Environmental Working Group (EWG) Guides

The Environmental Working Group is a nonprofit organization that empowers consumers to live healthier lives in a healthier environment. One of the organization's flagship initiatives is the publication of annual guides that rank fruits and vegetables based on their pesticide contamination levels. These guides provide consumers with valuable information about which produce items are most and least likely to contain pesticide residues, allowing them to make choices that minimize exposure to potentially harmful chemicals.

The "Dirty Dozen" and "Clean Fifteen" guides are two prominent resources offered by the EWG. The "Dirty Dozen" identifies the twelve produce items with the highest pesticide residues, while the "Clean Fifteen" highlights the fifteen items with the lowest pesticide residues. By consulting these guides, consumers can prioritize purchasing organic or pesticide-free options for the "Dirty Dozen" and feel more confident about choosing conventionally grown options for the "Clean Fifteen."

Benefits of EWG Guides
The EWG guides offer several benefits to consumers seeking to make informed choices about their food purchases. By highlighting which produce items are most and least contaminated with pesticides, these guides enable consumers to reduce their exposure to potentially harmful chemicals and minimize associated health risks. Additionally, the guides empower consumers to support sustainable farming practices by choosing organic or pesticide-free options whenever possible, thereby incentivizing agricultural methods prioritizing

environmental and human health.

Sustainable Seafood Guides

Concerns about overfishing and the depletion of marine resources have led to growing interest in sustainable seafood options. Sustainable Seafood Guides, such as the Monterey Bay Aquarium's Seafood Watch, provide consumers with valuable information about which seafood choices are environmentally responsible and which should be avoided due to overfishing or unsustainable harvesting practices. These guides typically categorize seafood into different rankings, ranging from "Best Choices" to "Avoid," based on population status, fishing methods, and habitat impacts.

Consumers can make informed decisions about which seafood products to purchase by consulting Sustainable Seafood Guides. This reduces demand for overexploited species and supports fisheries that prioritize sustainable practices. In this way, these guides play a crucial role in promoting the long-term health of marine ecosystems and ensuring the availability of seafood for future generations.

Community Supported Agriculture

Community-supported agriculture programs offer consumers a direct connection to local farmers and agricultural producers, allowing them to purchase fresh, seasonal produce directly from the source. In a CSA arrangement, consumers typically pay a subscription fee or membership dues to regularly receive a share of the farm's harvest. This model provides consumers access to fresh, locally grown produce and fosters a sense of community and support for small-scale, sustainable agriculture.

CSA programs reconnect consumers with the land and the people who produce their food, offering a transparent and direct alternative to conventional food distribution systems. By participating in a CSA, consumers can support local farmers, reduce the environmental impact of food transportation, and enjoy the benefits of seasonal eating. In many ways, CSA programs echo traditional agricultural practices, prioritizing community involvement, environmental stewardship, and the sustainable use of natural resources.

Conclusion: Reclaiming The Hunter's Path

Hunting has transcended mere sustenance throughout human history, embodying a profound connection with nature. From the early human traditions of tracking and hunting games to the modern-day pursuit of sustainably sourced foods, the essence of hunting endures in our quest for nourishment that honors nature and our bodies.

As we reflect on the journey from ancient to contemporary hunting practices, it becomes clear that the hunter's ethos has evolved alongside humanity's understanding of ethical sourcing, sustainability, and informed decision-making. Our ancestors, deeply attuned to their environments, navigated the natural world with reverence and respect, shaping their hunting practices to harmonize with the rhythms of wildlife and ecosystems.

Today, the spirit of the hunter lives on in the choices we make as consumers. Armed not with spears and arrows but with knowledge and awareness, we venture into supermarkets and farmers' markets, seeking foods that nourish us while upholding ethical and responsible principles and practices. The rise of certifications and labels, such as Fair Trade and USDA Organic, serves as progressive tracking signs, guiding us toward products that align with our values and beliefs.

The next chapter, "The Gatherer's Garden," will uncover the wealth of possibilities for nourishment within plant-based foods. Just as our ancestors foraged wild greens and cultivated backyard gardens, we will explore how to reconnect with these primitive practices and bring them into our current nutritional practices.

CHAPTER 3: THE GATHERER'S GARDEN

*Introduction: The Ancient
Roots of Foraging*

Foraging, gathering sustenance from the land, is a timeless art tracing back to ancient practices that once formed the backbone of human subsistence. It is a practice intricately intertwined with our ancestors' ecological literacy and survival skills. In its current iteration, the art and science of foraging demand a nuanced understanding of local flora, the nutritional value of wild edibles, and the seasonal rhythms in which they thrive. This knowledge empowers contemporary foragers to sustainably harvest plants that are not only rich in essential nutrients but also integral to local ecosystems. Ethical foraging practices ensure that one only takes what is needed, avoids overharvesting, and promotes the growth of plant populations by, for example, leaving enough berries to seed and not uprooting plants completely.

Foraging was indispensable to our ancestors, providing vital nutrients and medicinal plants from the natural environment. Modern foraging requires a deep understanding of local ecosystems, emphasizing ethical practices to ensure the sustainability of wild resources. This chapter celebrates the resilience of ancient traditions, highlighting their continued importance in fostering ecological harmony.

Challenges And Modern Adaptations

The popularity of foraging has brought about many challenges threatening this age-old practice. One of the most pressing challenges is the rampant overharvesting of trendy wild edibles fueled by commercial interests and culinary fads. For example, the popularity of foraged mushrooms has led to increased pressure on wild mushroom populations, risking their depletion and disrupting delicate forest ecosystems.

This unchecked exploitation of wild resources poses grave threats to biodiversity and the health of natural habitats. As certain species are overharvested, the delicate balance of ecosystems is disrupted, leading to cascading effects throughout the food source web. For instance, removing certain plant species may impact the availability of food and habitat for local wildlife, leading to declines in biodiversity.

Furthermore, the influx of novice foragers, eager to explore nature's bounty but needing more proper knowledge and experience, exacerbates these issues. Their well-intentioned but uninformed foraging expeditions can inadvertently damage fragile plant communities, disturb soil structures, and contribute to habitat degradation. For example, trampling through sensitive habitats or improperly harvesting plants can disrupt ecological processes and degrade the overall health of ecosystems.

In response to these pressing challenges, innovative solutions have emerged to preserve the essence of foraging while mitigating its negative impacts. One such adaptation is cultivating "forager's gardens," which offer a practical and sustainable approach to sourcing edible plants at home. These gardens are meticulously designed to mimic the diversity and complexity of wild ecosystems, cultivating native species that are nourishing for humans and beneficial for local flora and fauna.

For instance, a forager's garden may include native herbs like wild garlic and sorrel and edible flowers like violets and nasturtiums. These plants provide a steady supply of fresh, nutrient-rich foods and support local pollinators and beneficial insects. By embracing the concept of 'wildcrafting' within controlled environments, individuals can ensure a sustainable food source while minimizing their ecological footprint.

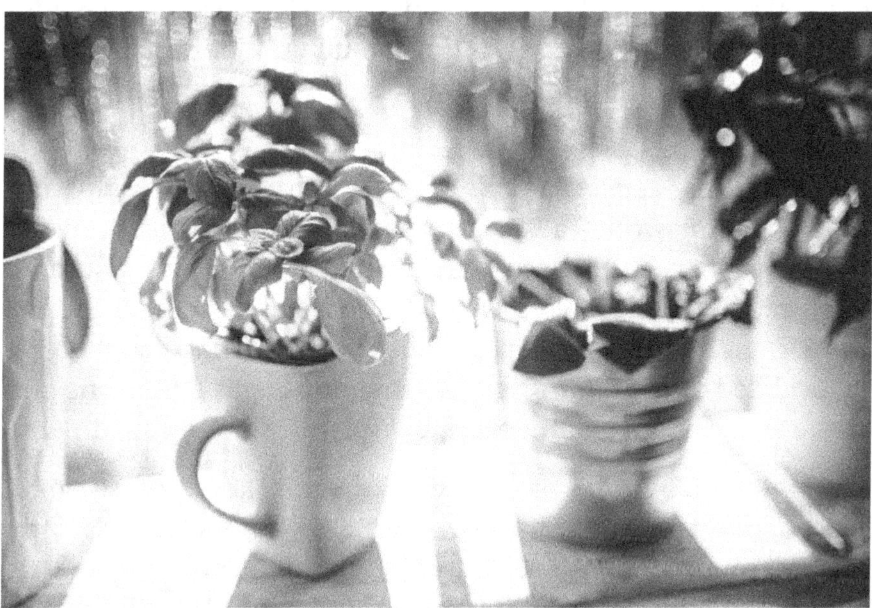

Moreover, forager's gardens serve as immersive educational tools, reconnecting individuals with the natural world and fostering a deeper appreciation for the interconnectedness of all living beings. Through hands-on gardening experiences, individuals gain a greater understanding of the ecological relationships that sustain life on Earth and the importance of responsible stewardship of natural resources.

Community Supported Agriculture

Community-supported agriculture represents a contemporary manifestation of the age-old practice of foraging. It seamlessly blends tradition with modernity to cultivate a deeper connection between consumers and the land. Through CSA programs, individuals can directly engage with local farms, forging meaningful relationships with the producers who nourish their communities.

By subscribing to CSAs, individuals gain access to a bounty of fresh, seasonal produce and become active participants in the sustainable agriculture movement. CSA subscribers play a vital role in preserving agricultural biodiversity and promoting environmentally conscious farming practices by supporting local farmers.

One compelling aspect of CSA participation is the reduction of carbon emissions associated with food transportation. Unlike supermarket produce, which often travels long distances before reaching the consumer, CSA produce is sourced locally, minimizing the environmental footprint of food distribution. This localized approach mitigates greenhouse gas emissions and fosters a sense of environmental stewardship among consumers.

Furthermore, CSA programs offer a diverse array of seasonal produce, reflecting the natural rhythms of the local ecosystem. From crisp apples in the fall to vibrant tomatoes in the summer, CSA subscribers experience the full spectrum of flavors and textures each season offers. This seasonal variety enriches culinary experiences and encourages a deeper appreciation for the cyclical nature of agricultural production.

In essence, CSA participation echoes the foraging ethos by reconnecting individuals with the origins of their food and fostering a sense of stewardship toward the land. Individuals nourish themselves and contribute to local food systems' vitality and resilience by supporting sustainable agriculture through CSA subscriptions.

Side Journey: Evolutionary Mutualism

The complex relationship between plants and animals has promoted a co-evolutionary trajectory where plants have developed ingenious strategies to ensure their survival and reproduction. This process has given rise to various nutrient-rich fruits, such as strawberries, blueberries, and raspberries, which rely on animals and humans to plant their seeds. Consumers are enticed by these fruits' vibrant colors and flavors and benefit from their essential vitamins and antioxidants. Subsequently, ingestion also promotes seed scatter via digestion and excretion.

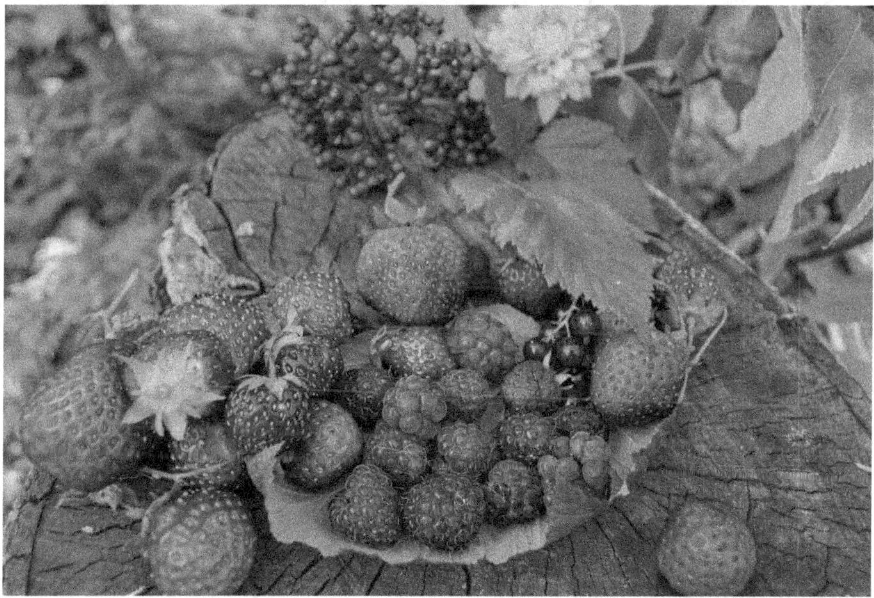

Beyond the realm of berries, numerous plants have embraced similar evolutionary tactics to encourage consumption and facilitate seed dispersal. Consider the ubiquitous apple, beloved for its crisp texture and sweet flavor. Apples have evolved to entice animals with their juicy flesh, enticing them to consume the fruit and scatter the seeds in new locations. Similarly, cherries offer a burst of tart sweetness that appeals to both animals and humans, ensuring the dispersal of their seeds.

In addition to fruits, nuts like chestnuts and walnuts have developed ingenious methods of seed dispersal. These nuts are encased in hard shells that protect the nutritious seeds within. Animals, including humans, crack open the shells to access the seeds, inadvertently dispersing them as they discard the inedible parts. This process ensures the propagation of these nut-bearing trees and contributes to the richness and diversity of forest ecosystems.

Furthermore, legumes such as peas and beans and root vegetables like carrots and beets have evolved to entice consumption through a combination of flavors and textures. Legumes offer a protein-rich source of sustenance, while root vegetables provide essential vitamins and minerals. Animals and humans alike are drawn to these nutrient-dense foods, unknowingly aiding in the dispersal of seeds as they consume the plant parts.

Through these evolutionary strategies, plants have forged mutually beneficial relationships with animals and humans, ensuring their propagation and contributing to the richness and resilience of ecosystems. These plants play a vital role in maintaining biodiversity and sustaining life on Earth by stimulating consumption and facilitating seed dispersal.

Conclusion: Reconnecting With Nature's Bounty

In conclusion, this chapter illuminates the profound insights gained from exploring the symbiotic relationship between humans, plants, and animals in the context of foraging and evolutionary mutualism. This exploration has uncovered pivotal realizations about our dietary habits and their long-term environmental impact.

Evolved foods that entice consumption support healthier eating and environmental stewardship. The nutrient-rich fruits and plants highlighted in this chapter nourish our bodies and contribute to ecosystems' richness and resilience. By aligning our diets with the rhythms of nature, we reduce our carbon footprint, support local ecosystems, and sustain traditional knowledge and practices. Choices such as participating in community-supported agriculture or cultivating a forager's garden at home are tangible ways to support sustainable and ethical farming practices, ensuring the continuation of biodiversity and traditional wisdom for future generations.

Ultimately, this chapter underscores the mutualism born of ancient evolutionary relationships and emphasizes our dietary choices' profound impact on our health and the environment. As stewards of the planet, it is incumbent upon us to make thoughtful decisions that honor these relationships and safeguard the health of our collective future. By embracing a sustainable, health-promoting dietary practice rooted in local, seasonal consumption and ethical farming; we can pave the way for a brighter, more resilient world for generations to come.

Transitioning from the realm of foraging and plant-based nutrition, our journey now takes us into the wild, where we delve into the complexities of sourcing meats and fish in harmony with nature.

CHAPTER 4: WILD AT HEART—MEATS AND FISH

Introduction: The Primal Hunt

In the deep recesses of human history, hunting and fishing emerged as leisurely pursuits and as primal necessities for survival. Embedded within the fabric of human culture, these ancient practices connect us to our primal roots, offering insights into the nutritional wisdom of our ancestors. In this chapter, we journeyed through time, exploring the virtues of embracing wild meats and fish in present-day diets. By delving into the historical context, nutritional significance, sustainable practices, ethical dimensions, and practical guidance surrounding the consumption of wild game and fish, we aim to illuminate the multifaceted benefits of reconnecting with these natural food sources.

Historical Context And Nutritional Significance

Hunting and fishing have transcended mere survival tactics throughout history, evolving into regulated practices that sustain human populations and ecosystem health. From the earliest hunter-gatherer societies to current conservation efforts, the significance of these practices cannot be overstated.

Consider the Inuit people of the Arctic, whose traditional diet consists primarily of wild-caught fish and marine mammals. For centuries, they have relied on the nutrient-rich bounty of the sea to sustain their communities, recognizing the unparalleled nutritional advantages of wild-caught seafood. Species such as salmon, cod, and halibut are prized for their abundance of omega-3 fatty acids, essential for brain health and cardiovascular function. By embracing a diet rich in these omega-3s, the Inuit people have thrived in one of the harshest environments on Earth, underscoring the nutritional significance of wild-caught fish.

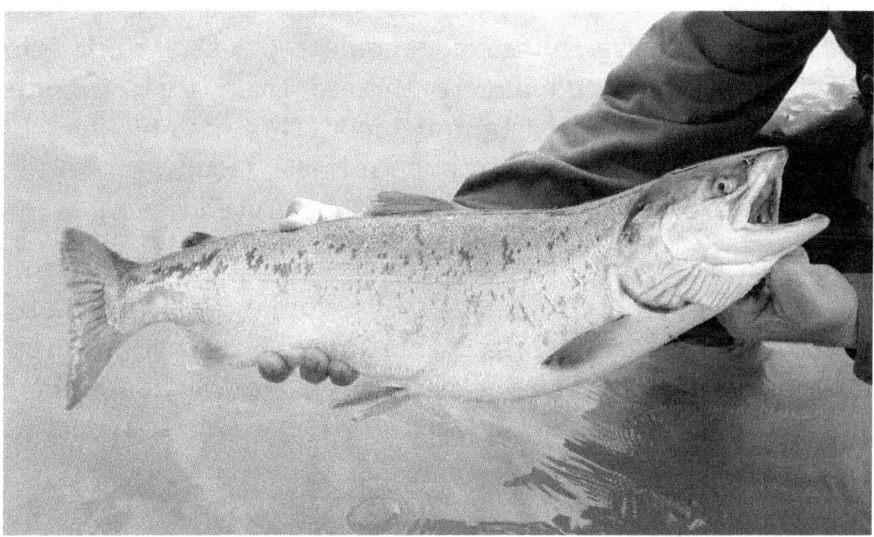

Similarly, indigenous tribes across the Americas have long revered the bounty of wild game as a cornerstone of their diets. For example, the Cherokee people of the southeastern United States traditionally hunted deer, elk, and wild turkey, recognizing the lean protein and essential nutrients these animals provided. By consuming these wild meats, they maintained robust health and vitality, free from the additives and contaminants in modern industrial agriculture.

In contrast to their wild counterparts, farmed meats and fish often contain antibiotics, hormones, and other synthetic additives that compromise their nutritional integrity. This stark contrast underscores the importance of embracing wild-caught options, which offer a more natural and health-promoting alternative. For instance, wild-caught salmon, prized for its rich flavor and vibrant color, contains higher levels of omega-3 fatty acids compared to its farmed counterpart. Wild game such as venison and bison are renowned for their lean protein content, providing a nutrient-dense option for those seeking optimal health.

Furthermore, the absence of antibiotics and hormones in wild-caught game and fish underscores their purity and wholesomeness. Unlike farmed animals, which are often subjected to intensive confinement and prophylactic antibiotic use, wild-caught specimens are free to roam their natural habitats, feeding on their natural diets. This natural lifestyle translates to healthier, more robust animals, resulting in meat and fish that are delicious and free from harmful additives.

The historical context and nutritional significance of hunting and fishing highlight the timeless wisdom of our ancestors, who understood the intrinsic value of wild-caught foods. By embracing these natural options in our diets, we honor their legacy and nourish our bodies with the wholesome goodness of nature's bounty.

Sustainable Practices: Modern Hunting And Fishing

In today's world, sustainable hunting and fishing practices are more critical than ever in preserving wildlife populations and ecosystem integrity. While traditional methods have evolved with modern techniques, the core principles of conservation remain at the forefront.

One current example of sustainable hunting practices in managing deer populations in various regions. In areas where deer populations have become overabundant, carefully regulated hunting seasons are implemented to help control numbers and prevent ecosystem imbalances. Hunters adhere to strict quotas and harvest limits, ensuring that deer populations remain stable and healthy while minimizing ecological damage caused by overgrazing.

Similarly, sustainable fishing practices play a vital role in maintaining the health of marine ecosystems. In commercial fisheries, catch limits, size restrictions, and seasonal closures are implemented to prevent overfishing and protect vulnerable species. For example, in the Pacific Northwest, managing salmon populations involves closely monitoring spawning runs and implementing fishing restrictions to ensure enough fish can reach their spawning grounds, thus safeguarding the species' future.

Moreover, the concept of "fair chase" principles extends beyond hunting to encompass ethical considerations in all aspects of outdoor recreation. For instance, catch-and-release fishing practices promote the conservation of fish populations by allowing anglers to enjoy the thrill of the sport without depleting local fish stocks. Anglers are encouraged to use barbless hooks, handle fish carefully, and release them unharmed back into the water, ensuring fish populations' longevity for future generations.

In addition to government regulations, many hunting and fishing organizations and associations have adopted voluntary conservation initiatives to promote sustainable practices further. These initiatives may include habitat restoration projects, wildlife monitoring programs, and educational outreach efforts to foster a deeper understanding of the importance of conservation among outdoor enthusiasts.

Overall, by adhering to sustainable hunting and fishing practices, hunters and anglers play a crucial role in preserving nature's delicate balance. Their efforts help safeguard the future of wildlife populations and ensure the continued enjoyment of outdoor recreation for generations to come.

The Ethical Dimension

Beyond the realm of sustenance, hunting and fishing carry profound implications rooted in respect for nature and responsible consumption. Ethical hunters and anglers view their pursuits not as mere sports but as a sacred connection to the natural world, guided by principles of stewardship and reverence for life. Through their efforts in conservation and habitat restoration, they embody the symbiotic relationship between humanity and the environment, recognizing that the health of one is intricately intertwined with the health of the other. Thus, hunting and fishing represent both a means of sustenance and a pathway to ecological harmony and personal fulfillment.

Practical Guidance: Incorporating Wild Meats And Fish Into Modern Diets

Practical guidance is essential for individuals seeking to incorporate the nutritional bounty of wild game and fish into their daily diets. Whether you're a seasoned outdoor enthusiast or a curious novice, navigating the world of wild meats and fish requires a nuanced approach that maximizes their health benefits while honoring their natural flavors.

When selecting wild meats and fish, sourcing from local hunters, fish markets, and specialty stores is critical. These outlets offer diverse options, from venison and elk to trout and wild-caught salmon, ensuring freshness and quality. By supporting local suppliers, you access the freshest ingredients and contribute to the sustainability of wild populations and the preservation of traditional hunting and fishing practices.

Once you've acquired your wild meats and fish, it's time to unleash your culinary creativity. Simple recipes and preparation methods highlighting these foods' natural essence are the order of the day. Consider grilling a succulent venison steak seasoned with herbs and spices or pan-searing a filet of wild-caught trout with a squeeze of lemon and a sprinkle of sea salt. The key is to let the natural flavors of the meat or fish shine through, enhancing rather than overpowering their innate richness.

Those new to cooking wild game and fish must familiarize themselves with proper handling and cooking techniques. Unlike their farmed counterparts, wild meats and fish may have a more robust flavor profile and leaner texture, requiring a gentler touch in the kitchen. Marinating meats with acidic ingredients such as vinegar or citrus juice can help tenderize them while bringing fish in saltwater can enhance their moisture and flavor.

Experimenting with different cooking methods can also yield delicious results. For a light and delicate dish, try smoking venison or elk for a deep, smoky flavor or poaching wild-caught fish in a fragrant broth. Embrace the versatility of wild meats and fish by incorporating them into various cuisines, from hearty stews and soups to elegant seafood pasta dishes. And if you are not ready to cook your meats and seafood, you can adopt traditional practices such as dry brining, vacuum sealing, and freezing your foods until you are ready to prepare them for eating.

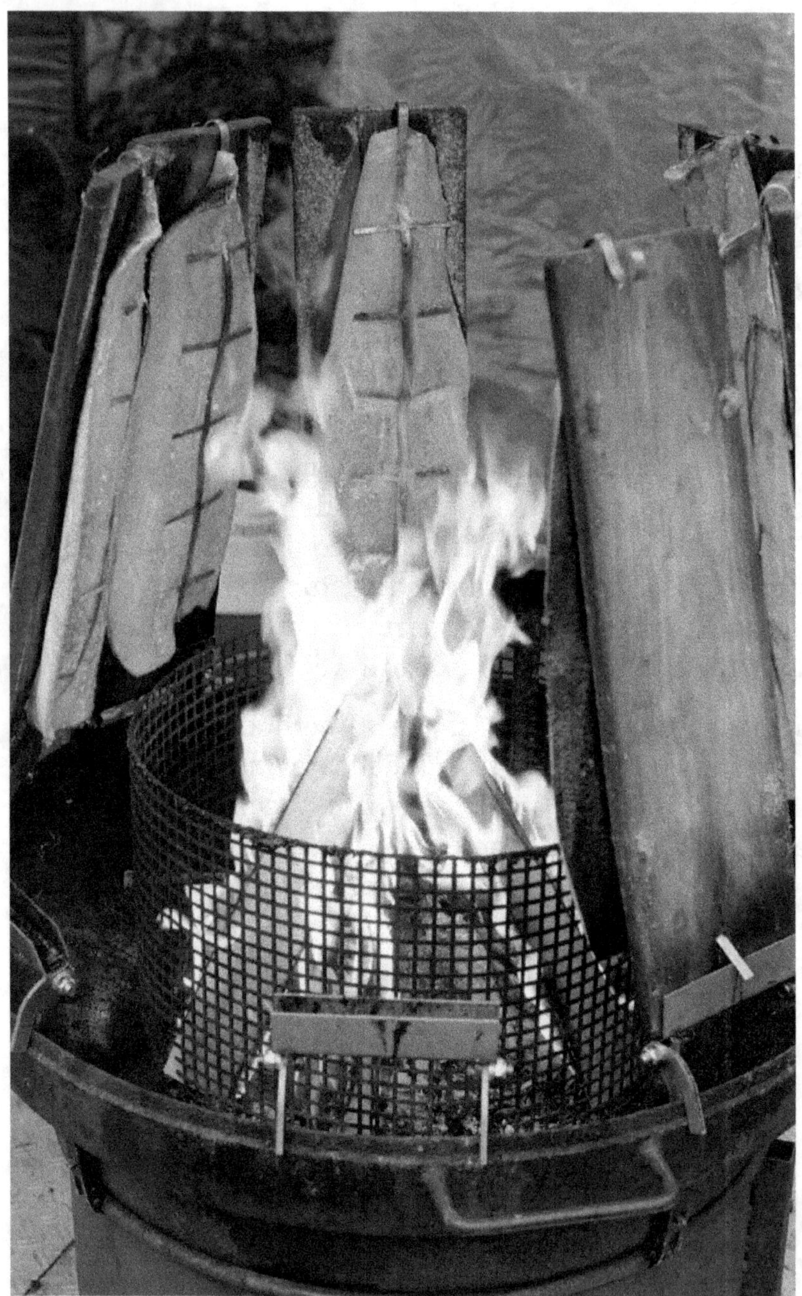

Above all, remember to savor the experience of preparing and enjoying wild game and fish. Whether you're gathered around the dinner table with family and friends or on a solo culinary adventure, each meal offers an opportunity to reconnect with the natural world and celebrate the richness of nature's offerings. So go ahead, embrace the nutritional bounty of wild meats and fish, and let your taste buds revel in the flavors of the great outdoors.

Conclusion: Reconnecting Through Responsible Choices

In conclusion, integrating wild game and fish into contemporary diets offers a pathway to reconnecting with ancestral dietary practices while promoting personal health and environmental sustainability. By embracing nutritional excellence and responsibility, individuals can make informed choices that resonate with the wisdom of the past and the needs of the future. As stewards of the land and waters, we can shape a world where our dietary choices nourish body and soul, ensuring a legacy of abundance for future generations.

As we reflect on the journey through the realm of wild meats and fish, we are reminded of the profound interconnectedness of all living beings. Our food choices hold the power to shape our bodies' health, our ecosystems' resilience, and the vitality of future generations. Just as we have delved into the nutritional wisdom of our ancestors through the consumption of wild game and fish, so too shall we now explore the healing powers of nature's botanical treasures. Let us reconnect with the remedies and medicinal marvels hidden within the forager's pharmacy that have sustained humanity for millennia.

CHAPTER 5:
THE FORAGER'S PHARMACY

Introduction: Nature's Healing Bounty

Every leaf and stem resides in a story of healing and wisdom —an ancestral knowledge passed down through generations. Our forebears were not just hunters and gatherers of food; they were adept at deciphering the language of plants to treat their ailments. Today, reconnecting with these wild medicinal plants enriches our health and sense of connection to the earth. This chapter ventures into the verdant world of medicinal wild plants, exploring their benefits and uses and reviving the lost art of natural remedies with a twist of engagement and safety.

The profound historical relationship between humans and medicinal plants is characterized by reverence, discovery, and healing. From the earliest days of human life, plants have been our steadfast companions, offering sustenance, shelter, and, perhaps most importantly, remedies for ailments. Ancient civilizations across the globe revered plants for their medicinal properties, cultivating a rich tradition of herbalism that persists to this day.

In every corner of the world, indigenous cultures developed deep knowledge systems surrounding the use of medicinal plants. From the Amazon rainforest to the plains of Africa and the mountains of Asia, traditional healers passed down generations of wisdom, unlocking the therapeutic potential of countless botanical species. These healers were practitioners and guardians of ancestral knowledge, intimately understanding the complex relationships between plants and human health.

The theme of "food as medicine" resonates deeply within these traditions, encapsulating the idea that what we consume has the power to heal and nourish us. In ancient wisdom, food was not merely sustenance; it was a form of medicine capable of preventing illness, restoring balance, and promoting vitality. This holistic approach to health emphasized the importance of a diverse and nutrient-rich diet abundant in fruits, vegetables, herbs, and spices.

Today, as we navigate the complexities of life and face an array of health challenges, the wisdom of our ancestors offers a beacon of guidance. The importance of revisiting traditional healing methods and incorporating them into contemporary lifestyles cannot be overstated. In an era dominated by pharmaceuticals and processed foods, there is a growing recognition of the need to reconnect with nature and embrace holistic approaches to health.

By revisiting traditional healing methods, we honor our ancestors' wisdom and tap into a rich reservoir of knowledge that offers profound insights into the art of healing. Incorporating these methods into contemporary lifestyles allows us to harness the therapeutic power of plants, fostering health and well-being in harmony with nature.

The historical relationship between humans and medicinal plants reminds us of our interconnectedness with the natural world. As we journey forward, let us draw upon the wisdom of the past to cultivate a future where food is not only sustenance but also medicine and traditional healing methods are valued as essential components of a holistic approach to health and wellness.

The Medicinal Power Of Plants

Plants have been foundational to medicine across civilizations and continue to play a crucial role today. Approximately 25% of drugs are derived directly or indirectly from plants. Rainforests, often called the "world's largest pharmacy," are particularly rich in medicinal plants, with less than 1% of tropical rainforest species having been studied for their medicinal potential, yet providing over 25% of the natural compounds used in drugs today (Jantan et al., 2015).

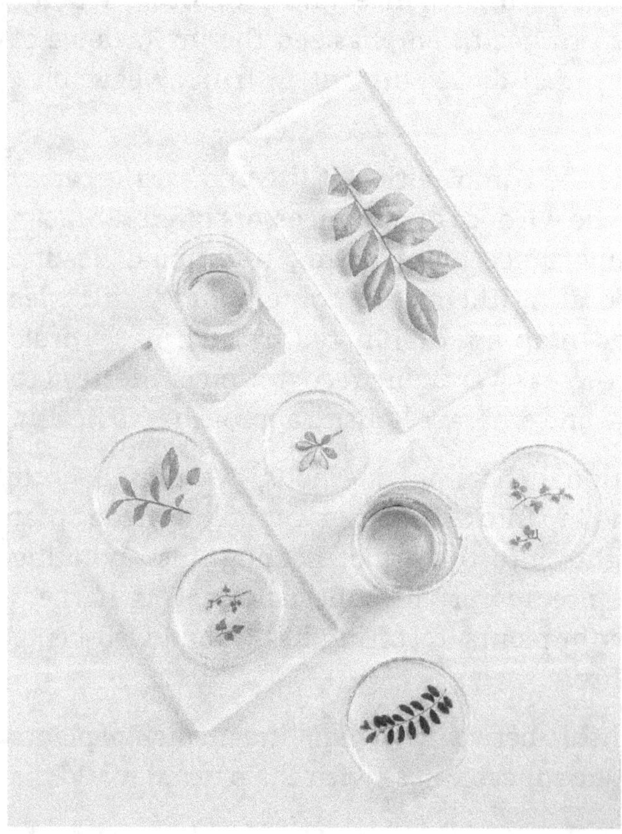

Plato's Influence on Contemporary

Nutritional Philosophy

Plato's adage, "Let food be thy medicine and medicine be thy food," reminds us of the intricate connection between our health and dietary choices. This profound philosophy transcends epochs, resonating with the fundamental truth that what we consume profoundly impacts our well-being. It underscores the notion that food is not merely fuel for our bodies but a potent source of healing and vitality.

This holistic perspective embraces the specific utilization of medicinal plants, recognizing them as nature's pharmacy brimming with bioactive compounds capable of preventing disease, restoring health, and offering therapeutic benefits. Within the rich tapestry of botanical diversity lie treasures revered for centuries for their remarkable healing properties.

Willow Bark—Nature's Aspirin

In the annals of herbal lore, willow bark is a testament to nature's ability to alleviate suffering. Renowned for its pain-relieving properties, willow bark has a storied history dating back to early practices. Civilizations spanning the globe, from the ancient Egyptians to the Native Americans, revered willow bark for its ability to ease pain and reduce fevers.

Central to its efficacy is salicin, a compound akin to aspirin, which imbues willow bark with its analgesic and anti-inflammatory prowess. Safely harnessing these benefits involves proper preparation methods, ensuring optimal extraction of the bark's medicinal constituents while mitigating potential side effects.

Lavender—The Soother

Lavender is a soothing balm for the body and soul in aromatic wonders. Its delicate blooms exude a fragrance that transcends mere scent, enveloping the senses in tranquility. Lavender's calming effects have been cherished for centuries, finding application in aromatherapy, tea preparation, and an array of cultural rituals.

Beyond its aromatic allure, lavender possesses therapeutic properties that soothe frayed nerves, alleviate stress, and promote relaxation. From ancient Egypt to medieval Europe, lavender has been esteemed for its ability to induce a sense of calm and serenity. Whether infused in a fragrant tea or diffused in an essential oil, lavender continues to enchant and heal across generations.

Echinacea—The Immune Booster

Amidst the expansion of medicinal flora, echinacea stands tall as a stalwart defender of immune health. Revered by indigenous cultures for centuries, echinacea has left an indelible mark on the landscape of traditional medicine. Its immune-boosting properties have been harnessed to ward off colds, flu, and other disorders, serving as a potent ally in the fight against illness.

Rich in bioactive compounds such as alkamides and polysaccharides, echinacea stimulates the immune system, enhancing its ability to combat pathogens and maintain health. From primitive healing traditions to contemporary herbalism, echinacea's legacy is a beacon of hope and resilience in uncertain times. With proper guidance, homemade remedies harnessing echinacea's immune-boosting prowess can be crafted, ensuring its therapeutic benefits are accessible to all.

Plants In The Modern Diet: Preventive Health

Incorporating medicinal plants into daily diets is an effective way to harness their health benefits. Many of these plants contain antioxidants, anti-inflammatory agents, and other phytochemicals that can help reduce the risk of chronic diseases such as cancer, diabetes, and heart disease. For example:

- **Turmeric**, with its active compound curcumin, is renowned for its anti-inflammatory and antioxidant properties.

- **Ginger** is widely used for its antiemetic properties, helping alleviate nausea and boasting anti-inflammatory effects.

- **Garlic** is known for its cardiovascular benefits, helping to lower blood pressure and cholesterol levels. These plants can be easily incorporated into diets through teas, spices in cooking, or as supplements, making the preventive aspects of health not only accessible but also simple to integrate into daily routines.

Juicing and Its Benefits: Celery as a Case Study

Juicing is a popular method to quickly consume a concentrated amount of vegetables' beneficial compounds. Celery juice, in particular, has gained popularity for its numerous health benefits. This is mainly due to its high levels of antioxidants and phytochemicals, such as vitamin C, beta carotene, and flavonoids. Celery also contains a compound called apigenin, an anti-inflammatory molecule that can help to reduce inflammation and blood pressure—moreover, juicing celery results in a high concentration of these beneficial compounds in an easily digestible form, making it a practical choice for daily health maintenance.

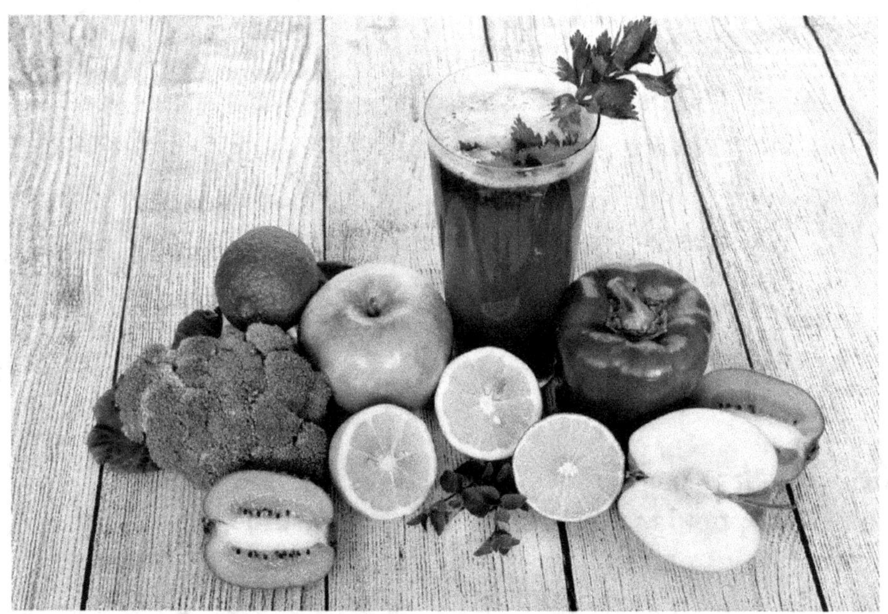

Practical Applications And Safety Guidelines

Each plant profile includes safe preparation techniques, from teas and tinctures to poultices. Following step-by-step processes to extract maximum benefits is essential, ensuring these methods are accessible to beginners and seasoned foragers alike. Safety is paramount when dealing with medicinal plants. The reader must be educated on identifying correct plant species, understanding proper dosages, and knowing potential interactions with conventional medications, which are crucial for safe usage.

Conclusion: Embracing Plant-Based Wisdom

Exploring the realm of medicinal plants allows us to experience a transformation that transcends physical well-being and delves into our connection with nature. By understanding the ancient wisdom encapsulated within medicinal flora leaves, roots, and blossoms, we develop deeper self-discovery and holistic healing.

Throughout this chapter, we have learned ways to integrate

the timeless knowledge of medicinal plants into our daily lives, forging a symbiotic relationship between human health, environmental stewardship, and cultural heritage. Through this integration, we not only cultivate healthier bodies but also contribute to the preservation of biodiversity and traditional wisdom.

As we bridge the wisdom of the past with the imperatives of modern health, we seed a healthier, more harmonious future. Let us heed the call to action, embracing the bounty of nature's pharmacy with open hearts and minds. By nurturing our bodies and the planet with the age-old wisdom of the forager's pharmacy, we pave the way for a world where health, sustainability, and cultural heritage intertwine seamlessly.

Having explored the profound insights offered by nature's pharmacy, our journey now takes us into the realm of data-driven dietary wisdom. In the upcoming chapter, "Decoding Diets with Data," we delve into the intersection of nutrition science and technology, uncovering the secrets to personalized dietary approaches tailored to individual health needs.

CHAPTER 6: DECODING DIETS WITH DATA

Introduction: The New Frontier of Nutritional Science

Data analytics and AI advancements are revolutionizing nutritional science by allowing researchers to integrate and analyze complex datasets. For example, integrating genomic databases with historical dietary records and real-time health data provides new insights into the relationship between genetics, diet, and health outcomes. As we stand on the brink of a new era in nutritional science, the integration of data analytics and artificial intelligence is heralding unprecedented advancements that promise to reshape our understanding of diet and health. Traditionally, nutritional studies have relied on controlled experiments and epidemiological surveys to draw connections between dietary patterns and health outcomes. In the current era of big data, the complexity of human biology, including diverse variables influencing nutrition—from genetics to lifestyle—has often left researchers grappling with data as vast as it is intricate.

Moreover, AI's capability to integrate and interpret data from diverse sources has enabled robust predictions of how historical eating habits have shaped modern health. Researchers now use AI to dig into anthropological data, extracting dietary insights from rediscovered bones, teeth, and even the residues found in millennia-old cooking vessels. These studies detail how our ancestors' diets influenced their health and evolution, offering critical lessons for contemporary nutritional science. For instance, a recent study utilized machine learning to analyze dietary data from thousands of individuals across multiple continents. Researchers identified dietary patterns correlated with reduced risk of chronic diseases, such as Type 2 Diabetes and cardiovascular disorders (Morgenstern et al., 2021). These patterns were then cross-referenced with genetic markers, providing insights into how individual genetic variations affect dietary needs and health outcomes.

This burgeoning field, called 'nutritional informatics,' is poised to become a cornerstone of health sciences. It combines the rigors of empirical research with the innovative potential of information technology, transforming how we understand the building blocks of our diet and their impact on our bodies. As we continue to navigate this new frontier, the promise of AI in unlocking the secrets of nutritional science is not just exciting—it's revolutionary. This chapter will explore these advancements in-depth, examining their potential and the challenges they bring to the forefront of health and dietary science.

The Rise Of Nutritional Informatics

Nutritional informatics is a burgeoning field that leverages information technology to collect, analyze, and disseminate dietary data. For example, the National Institutes of Health (NIH) supports the FoodData Central database, which compiles data from various studies to provide comprehensive information on food nutrients. The FoodData Central database exemplifies the transformative potential of nutritional informatics in advancing public health and well-being. By harnessing the power of data-driven insights, this innovative resource enables stakeholders across sectors to promote optimal nutrition, prevent disease, and improve health outcomes for individuals and communities.

One notable example of FoodData Central's utility is its role in elucidating the nutritional profiles of staple foods. For instance, researchers can access detailed information on the macronutrient and micronutrient content of common foods such as fruits, vegetables, grains, and proteins. This data not only aids in assessing the nutritional adequacy of diets but also informs dietary recommendations tailored to specific populations or health conditions.

Moreover, FoodData Central facilitates comparative analyses across different food items, allowing researchers to explore variations in nutrient content based on factors such as processing methods, geographical origin, and agricultural practices. For instance, studies may examine how cooking methods affect vitamin retention in vegetables or how soil composition influences the mineral content of crops.

Beyond its utility in research, FoodData Central is a valuable resource for healthcare professionals seeking to educate patients about optimal nutrition. By accessing the database's user-friendly interface, clinicians can retrieve accurate and up-to-date information on the nutrient composition of foods, facilitating personalized dietary counseling and meal planning.

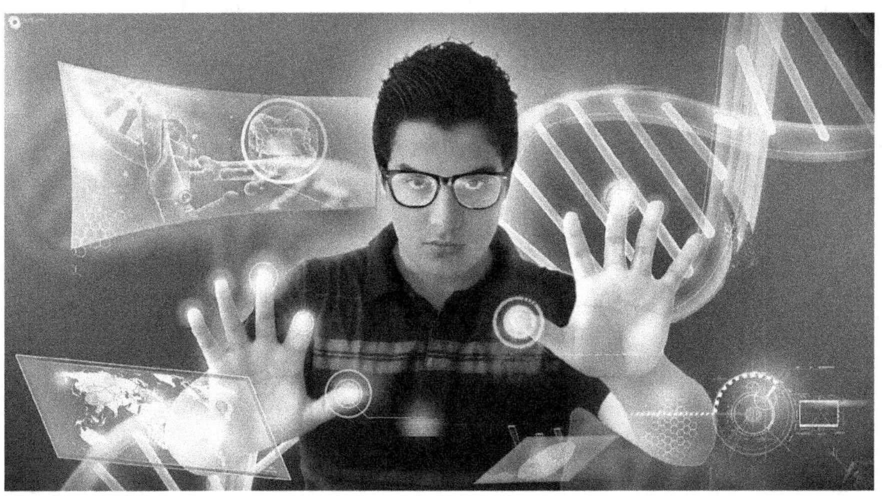

Case Studies: Rediscovering Primitive Diets

AI also revolutionizes our understanding of past human diets through sophisticated data analysis. Recent advancements demonstrate AI's potential to recreate historical dietary patterns accurately. For instance, AI's ability to interpret complex data from diverse sources allows researchers to deduce past food consumption comprehensively. A notable application is its use in analyzing isotopic data to reconstruct the diets of ancient populations. This method provides insights into the types of plants and animals consumed, offering a clearer picture of early human nutrition. Such studies suggest reevaluating historical diet compositions, potentially altering our understanding of early agricultural practices and societal organization.

Recent research led by the University of Wyoming provides compelling evidence that early Andeans primarily subsisted on a plant-based diet (Chen et al., 2024), revolutionizing our understanding of early human diets in South America. Analyzing remains from the Wilamaya Patjxa and Soro Mik'aya Patjxa sites in Peru, the study revealed an unexpected dietary composition of 80% plant matter and only 20% meat, challenging the long-held notion of 'hunter-gatherers.' By employing methods such as isotope chemistry and statistical modeling, researchers uncovered that these early humans heavily relied on tubers and other plant materials, which has significant implications for our understanding of early agricultural practices and dietary preferences in the Andes. This groundbreaking research shifts the narrative from a meat-centric to a plant-dominant diet among ancient Andean populations, reshaping our historical perspective on their subsistence strategies.

Ai In Personalized Nutrition

Recently, there has been a trend toward hyper-personalized nutrition, where AI is crucial in transforming a vast array of health data into actionable, personalized eating plans. This improves individual health outcomes and paves the way for a future where diet-related diseases can be preemptively managed through tailored nutrition.

Nutrigenomix harnesses the power of DNA analysis to provide personalized nutrition advice. By analyzing an individual's genetic profile, Nutrigenomix crafts tailored dietary strategies to mitigate health risks associated with obesity and Type 2 Diabetes. While the direct use of AI is not explicitly mentioned, the potential integration of AI could enhance the accuracy and effectiveness of these genetic analyses by quickly processing large datasets to identify patterns and predict health outcomes. This would lead to more precise nutritional recommendations based on genetic predispositions.

The ZOE project represents a significant step forward in personalized nutrition by integrating blood glucose monitoring, gut microbiome analysis, and individual dietary habits. This approach has shown that people respond differently to the same foods, underlining the necessity for personalized dietary plans. The application of AI in ZOE could further refine these insights by analyzing real-time data streams from various biometric sources to dynamically tailor dietary recommendations that optimize metabolic health for each individual.

Finally, integrating AI with biometric monitoring technologies marks a new era in personalized nutrition. Real-time tracking devices that monitor metrics like blood glucose levels and gut microbiome conditions are now being enhanced with AI capabilities. This technology can process physiological data to recommend personalized diets, adapting to an individual's unique food responses. This mirrors the old practice of adjusting diets based on environmental and seasonal factors but with modern technological sophistication, making it a contemporary revival of adaptive eating practices tailored to personal health needs.

Technology Meets Tradition

IBM's AI for Good initiative has significantly improved the preservation of traditional food knowledge through artificial intelligence. The program works collaboratively with indigenous communities to digitize many traditional plant uses. This includes documenting medicinal, culinary, and cultural practices tied to specific plants, effectively creating a vast database that serves as a reservoir of knowledge and a tool for biodiversity conservation and cultural heritage preservation. Digitization of traditional knowledge helps identify and conserve biodiversity. It ensures that information about endangered plant species and their unique uses are preserved and shared, promoting sustainable practices crucial for ecological health. This digital archive aids in safeguarding cultural identities and histories, making them accessible to future generations and helping maintain the diversity of cultural practices worldwide.

Google AI has used machine learning to analyze environmental data and satellite images, which helps identify optimal areas for reintegrating native plants into modern agricultural practices. This project supports the sustainable cultivation of traditional crops by identifying optimal planting areas and supporting biodiversity.

By analyzing satellite imagery and environmental data, Google AI's project identifies the best areas for planting native crops. This integration of advanced technology into agriculture not only aids in preserving traditional agricultural knowledge but also enhances food security and sustainability. The project contributes to ecological balance by promoting the growth of native plants, which are often more adapted to local conditions and require fewer agricultural inputs.

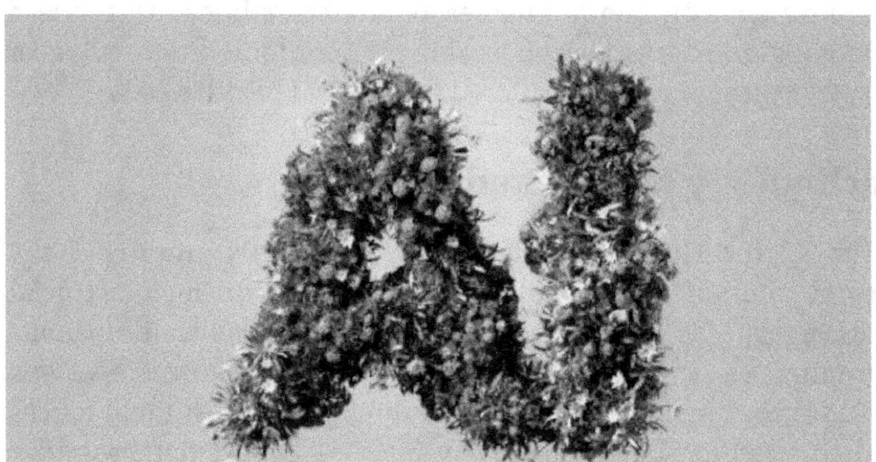

Challenges and Ethical Considerations

The advancement of technology also introduces new challenges, such as the risk of data bias and privacy concerns associated with collecting and analyzing dietary data. The European Union's General Data Protection Regulation (GDPR) is an example framework aiming to protect personal data and privacy, which impacts how researchers and tech companies must handle dietary data (GOV.UK, 2018). Ethical considerations are paramount in ensuring global, equitable access to AI-driven nutritional advice.

Conclusion: Future Directions and Innovations

IBM and Google's initiatives illustrate how AI can bridge the gap between traditional knowledge and present-day technology, ensuring that valuable historical and cultural practices are preserved and integrated into contemporary applications. Approaches such as these contribute to conserving biodiversity and cultural heritage and offer practical solutions to current and future challenges in agriculture and medicine.

As AI technology progresses and continues to integrate deeper with all aspects of our daily lives, it is foreseeable that technology will be available via our watches or earbuds that will provide us with real-time dietary recommendations based on physiological data like blood sugar levels and metabolic rates. Furthermore, as global nutritional databases expand, so will AI's ability to provide crop or dietary plans and public health recommendations and address nutritional deficiencies individually and globally.

CHAPTER 7: THE DIGITAL HUNTER-GATHERER

Introduction: Adapting Ancient Practices for the Modern Age

In the vast expanse of the digital age, our fundamental connection to the sources of our sustenance is transforming as profoundly as the agricultural revolution. As our ancestors once roamed the wilds, expertly reading the land to sustain their communities, today's consumers navigate a virtual landscape, hunting and gathering information to make principled and health-conscious food choices. This adaptation uses digital tools to recreate ancient practices of sourcing nourishing food via principled practices. As we delve deeper into this chapter, we explore how these digital foraging practices represent a necessity and a conscious choice to reconnect with our primal roots in a world inundated with processed foods and disconnected eating habits.

Navigating The Digital Food Landscape

The transition from physical to digital foraging marks an evolution in how individuals procure food that aligns with their dietary and ethical preferences. Online platforms have become indispensable tools, enabling consumers to access information and resources to support their nutritional needs and values in the urban environment. Apps and websites have emerged as key facilitators in this transformation, allowing individuals to discover and procure local, organic, and wild foods. By leveraging these digital tools, foraging practices find relevance in contemporary contexts, bridging the gap between tradition and modernity.

The proliferation of mobile applications such as "Seasonal Food Guide" exemplifies this shift, empowering users to make informed choices about food purchases. These apps offer insights into the best times to buy produce locally for optimal freshness and provide valuable information on seasonal availability alongside recipes and storage recommendations. Thus, they streamline the process of making sustainable food choices, making it more accessible and effortless for consumers.

The Role Of Ai In Fostering Sustainable Consumer Practices

AI technologies are pivotal in reshaping the dietary landscape by offering personalized nutritional guidance and fostering sustainable consumer behaviors. Platforms like Nutrigenomix leverage individual genetic profiles to deliver customized dietary recommendations, optimizing personal well-being and promoting mindful consumption. This tailored approach has the potential to curtail overconsumption and minimize waste, aligning with principles of sustainable living.

Projects like ZOE utilize AI algorithms to analyze data from blood glucose monitoring and gut microbiome assessments, devising personalized dietary plans that enhance metabolic health. This nuanced understanding of individual dietary responses can engender more sustainable eating habits as consumers learn to adapt their diets based on their body's unique requirements, reducing unnecessary consumption and waste generation.

AI and Biometric Technologies: Pioneering Personalized Nutrition

Integrating AI with biometric monitoring devices represents a significant leap forward in personalized nutrition. Wearable gadgets that track physiological responses to dietary intake furnish invaluable data for AI systems to process, enabling the provision of real-time dietary recommendations. This optimizes individual health outcomes and echoes dietary practices rooted in adaptability to seasonal and environmental factors. This fusion of cutting-edge technology with age-old wisdom exemplifies a sophisticated approach to minimizing food waste and maximizing dietary efficiency, illustrating how traditional principles can be revitalized through innovation.

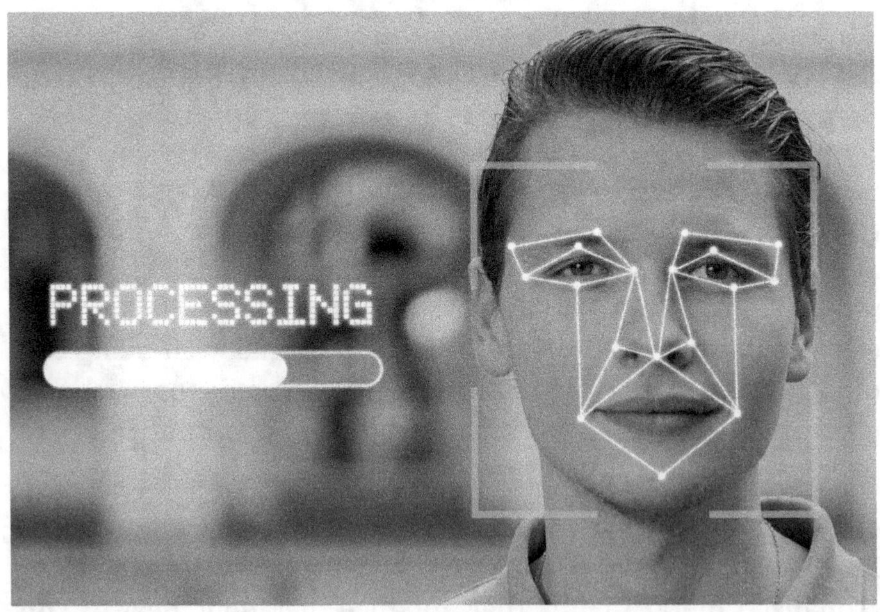

Profiles Of Digital Foragers

Digital foragers using technology to enhance food-sourcing practices are reminiscent of early foraging traditions. Examples include urban gardeners utilizing apps for produce swapping and families participating in Community Supported Agriculture programs. It highlights initiatives like the GrownBy app, which directly connects consumers with local farmers, fostering community bonds and supporting sustainable agriculture. By bypassing traditional retail channels, such platforms empower farmers and ensure a stable supply of fresh produce, particularly during crises like the COVID-19 pandemic. This integration of technology with traditional practices evolves the concept of foraging, promoting sustainable consumption and bolstering the resilience of local food systems.

Challenges And Limitations

Digital foragers face challenges related to digital literacy, technology access, and online information reliability. Potential pitfalls in digital foraging often focus on the commodification of traditional knowledge or the risk of exacerbating social inequalities through technology-access disparities.

Empowering Consumers Through Education And Technology

Various educational initiatives and tools aim to empower consumers to become adept digital foragers. These include tutorials on sustainability assessment of food sources and workshops on utilizing digital tools for food procurement. It discusses the potential of AI and machine learning to personalize food-sourcing recommendations based on individual health data and environmental impacts. Additionally, it highlights initiatives like "Code for America," which develops apps to assist low-income families in locating farmers' markets accepting food stamps, thus democratizing access to nutritious food. Educational programs, such as university online courses, further equip consumers with skills to understand food labels, assess quality, and make informed nutritional choices. These are crucial for navigating food markets in line with health goals and ethical values.

Leveraging Digital Platforms for Seed Sharing and Knowledge Exchange

Social media platforms can effectively be used as digital commons. For social media groups interested in foraging, these platforms serve as hubs for exchanging seeds, sharing gardening tips, and discussing seed-saving techniques, thus enhancing community knowledge and connectivity.

Blockchain Technology for Transparent Supply Chains

Blockchain technology, particularly by companies like IBM, is being used to ensure transparency and accountability in food supply chains. With IBM Blockchain, stakeholders can access an immutable ledger tracking a product's journey from farm to table, enhancing supply chain visibility and management. IBM's Food Trust™ platform enhances traceability and efficiency, bolstering consumer confidence in food safety and verifying claims about organic or fair-trade practices. Additionally, AI is essential in optimizing local supply chains by analyzing consumer buying patterns and accurately forecasting demand, thus reducing food waste and promoting economic and environmental sustainability. Blockchain and AI technologies contribute to more intelligent, accountable, and efficient supply chains, fostering sustainable consumption practices and empowering informed consumer choices.

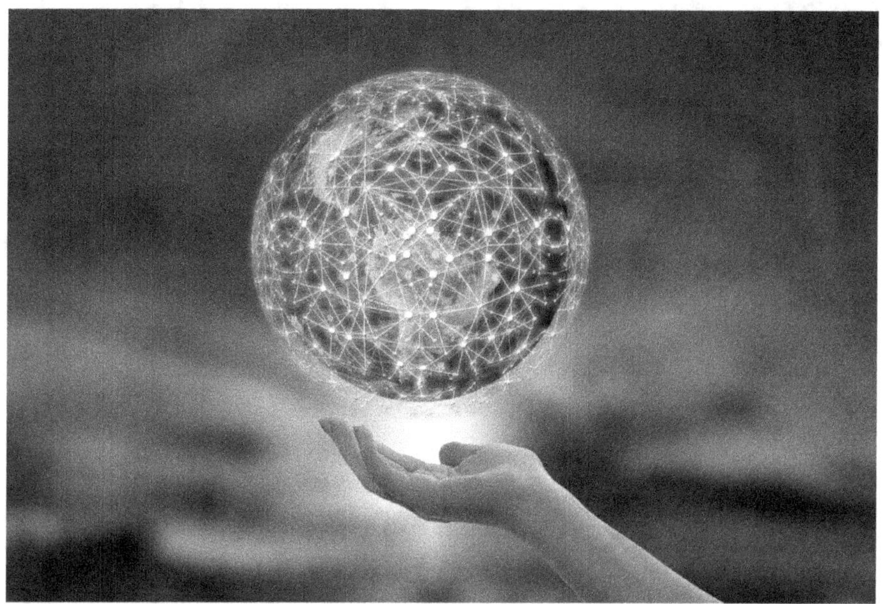

Conclusion: The Future Of Foraging

Integrating traditional foraging knowledge with cutting-edge technology preserves and enhances our relationship with the environment, promoting a balanced ecosystem and a healthier society. As digital tools become more sophisticated and widely accessible, they have the potential to revolutionize our food systems, making sustainable eating the norm rather than the exception.

Examples of smart devices like dietary tracking glasses and nutritional scanners showcase technologies that promise to offer immediate feedback on dietary choices and contribute to improved health outcomes. These technologies also have environmental benefits, such as reducing food waste and supporting sustainability. Furthermore, they have the potential to influence cultural norms around eating, promoting personalized nutrition and sustainable habits. In this chapter, we have emphasized transforming foraging into a technologically augmented practice, advocating for the continued embrace of these tools to foster informed and sustainable eating habits.

CHAPTER 8: AI IN AGRICULTURE— BRIDGING THE PAST AND FUTURE

*Introduction: The Essence
of Ritual in Eating*

In our fast-paced world, where convenience often takes precedence over connection, the importance of rituals in eating cannot be overstated. From the dawn of civilization, rituals have been intertwined with our food practices, shaping how we nourish our bodies and connect with nature, community, and cultural heritage. In this chapter, we delve into the transformative role of artificial intelligence in agriculture, exploring how it revolutionizes our approach to food production and sustainability and rekindles the ancient rituals that once defined our relationship with food.

Rituals, whether observed in the planting of crops, the harvesting of fruits, or the preparation of meals, have served as sacred threads weaving together the fabric of society. They offer a means of expressing gratitude to the earth for its bounty, honoring the toil of farmers, and fostering a sense of unity among communities. In the hustle and bustle of life, however, these rituals have often been relegated to the sidelines, overshadowed by the allure of convenience and efficiency.

Yet, as we stand at the crossroads of tradition and innovation, a renewed appreciation emerges for the timeless wisdom of these age-old rituals. With its unparalleled capacity for data analysis, predictive modeling, and automation, AI is not merely a tool for increasing yields or optimizing resource allocation but a catalyst for reconnecting with our agricultural heritage in profound and meaningful ways.

The Past Meets the Future: AI Reshaping Agricultural Practices

The journey of AI in agriculture is one marked by innovation, ingenuity, and a deep reverence for the wisdom of the past. Drawing inspiration from agricultural practices while harnessing the power of cutting-edge technology, AI is bridging the gap between tradition and contemporary in unprecedented ways.

Historically, agricultural rituals were deeply rooted in the rhythms of nature, guided by the cycles of the seasons and the wisdom passed down through generations. Today, AI algorithms are leveraging vast troves of data, from soil composition and weather patterns to crop yields and market trends, to optimize every facet of the agricultural process. By analyzing historical data and real-time inputs, AI systems can predict optimal planting times, identify areas of pest infestation or nutrient deficiency, and even automate the operation of farm machinery with precision and efficiency.

Moreover, AI facilitates a renaissance of sustainable agricultural practices, echoing the ethos of stewardship and harmony with nature espoused by our ancestors. Using drones equipped with multi-spectral imaging cameras, for instance, farmers can monitor crop health and soil moisture levels with unprecedented accuracy, enabling targeted interventions that minimize environmental impact and maximize resource efficiency.

The Human Touch: Cultivating Connection in the Digital Age

Amidst the expanding array of sensors, algorithms, and drones populating the agricultural landscape, it is crucial to maintain sight of the human element at the heart of food production. While AI can optimize processes and increase yields, human ingenuity, empathy, and creativity ultimately determine the success of agricultural endeavors.

In this sense, AI serves not as a replacement for human labor but as a complement, amplifying our capabilities and enabling us to achieve feats once thought impossible. Beyond its role in optimizing agricultural practices, AI enables farmers to cultivate deeper connections with the land and their communities. By providing personalized recommendations and tailored solutions, AI facilitates sustainable land management practices that promote soil health, biodiversity, and ecosystem resilience. Moreover, AI-powered platforms and tools foster collaboration and knowledge sharing among farmers, enabling them to learn from each other's experiences, adapt to changing conditions, and collectively address common challenges. By automating repetitive tasks and providing insights gleaned from vast datasets, AI empowers farmers to focus on what truly matters: nurturing the land, fostering community, and preserving the rich tapestry of agricultural traditions that have sustained us for millennia.

Nourishing Body, Mind, and Soul

In the age of AI, the ritual of eating takes on new dimensions, infused with the spirit of innovation and reverence for the past. As we harness the transformative power of artificial intelligence to reshape the agricultural landscape, let us not forget the lessons of our ancestors: that food is more than mere sustenance—it is a sacred bond that unites us with the earth, with each other, and with generations yet unborn.

By embracing the wisdom of the past and the possibilities of the future, we can cultivate a more sustainable, resilient, and interconnected food system that nourishes our bodies, minds, and souls. In this union of tradition and technology, we find hope for a world where the ritual of eating is not just a means to an end but a celebration of life itself.

Historical Perspectives On Eating Rituals

Throughout history, food rituals have played a significant role in shaping cultural identities and fostering community bonds. From the ceremonial feasts of Native American tribes to the elaborate tea ceremonies of Japan, these rituals have reflected a deep reverence for food and its role in spiritual, social, and cultural life. However, as societies have undergone industrialization, technological advancements, and urbanization, there has been a notable shift toward faster, less mindful eating practices. This chapter explores the changes in food rituals brought about by industrialization, noting the erosion of traditional practices and the emergence of convenience-oriented consumption habits.

Traditional Food Rituals

In traditional societies, food rituals were deeply ingrained in daily life, serving as occasions for celebration, gratitude, and connection with the natural world. For example, Native American tribes engaged in ritual dances and feasts to honor the spirits and express gratitude for bountiful harvests. These communal gatherings provided sustenance, strengthened social bonds, and preserved cultural heritage. Similarly, in Japan, the tea ceremony (*Chanoyu*) was a meticulously choreographed ritual that elevated drinking tea to an art form. Participants engaged in precise movements and gestures, fostering mindfulness and promoting a deep appreciation for life's aesthetic and spiritual dimensions.

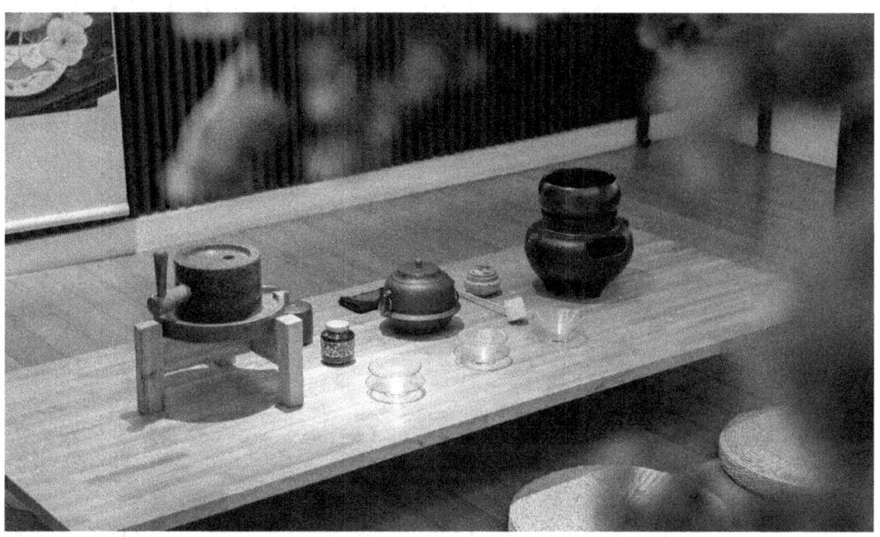

Impact of Industrialization: Disconnection From Food Sources

The shift towards industrialization revolutionized every aspect of the food system, from cultivation to consumption. Agriculture underwent significant transformations with the introduction of machinery, chemical fertilizers, and pesticides. These innovations boosted crop yields and allowed the large-scale production of staple foods like wheat, corn, and rice. As a result, food became more abundant and affordable, improving many's living standards. Transportation played a crucial role in connecting distant food-producing regions with urban centers. The development of railways, refrigerated trucks, and air freight facilitated the long-distance transport of perishable goods. This meant people could access a wider variety of foods year-round, regardless of seasonal availability or geographic location.

Consequently, diets diversified, incorporating ingredients from around the globe. Food processing technologies also underwent significant advancements during the industrial era.

Canning, freezing, and dehydration techniques emerged, extending the shelf life of foods and making them more convenient to store and transport. Additionally, innovations in packaging, such as the introduction of cardboard boxes and plastic wrap, further contributed to the preservation and distribution of food products. The proliferation of processed and convenience foods reshaped eating habits and food culture. With the rise of urbanization, people increasingly gravitated towards quick and easy meal options that required minimal preparation.

Traditional food rituals, such as the family dinner, gradually declined as hectic schedules and individualized lifestyles became the norm. Instead of sitting down for a leisurely meal, many opted for on-the-go eating, grabbing fast food or microwavable dinners to accommodate busy schedules. This shift towards convenience also had profound implications for health and nutrition. Processed foods often contain high levels of sugar, salt, and unhealthy fats, leading to an increase in diet-related illnesses such as obesity, diabetes, and cardiovascular disease. Moreover, the commodification of food production led to the prioritization of profit over sustainability and nutritional value, resulting in environmental degradation and loss of biodiversity.

Industrialization and urbanization have also contributed to a growing disconnection between food sources and the natural world. With the rise of supermarkets and fast-food chains, many people have become detached from the origins of their food and the processes involved in its production. As a result, mealtime has been devalued as a space for social bonding, relaxation, and cultural expression. Instead of gathering around a table to share a meal with loved ones, people often eat alone or on the run, prioritizing convenience over mindful consumption.

However, alongside these challenges, there have been efforts to reclaim and revive traditional food practices in response to the homogenization of food culture. The slow food movement, for instance, advocates for preserving local culinary traditions, sustainable farming practices, and promoting community-based food systems. Similarly, there has been a growing interest in organic farming, farmers' markets, and farm-to-table dining experiences, reflecting a desire for fresher, healthier, and more ethically sourced food options.

Modern Rituals And Technology

Technology presents an opportunity to revive and reinvent food rituals in response to today's fast-paced, disconnected eating habits. Innovations such as apps promoting slow-cooking recipes or community cooking events leverage technology to foster engagement and connection around food. Examples include 'EatWith,' an app facilitating communal dining experiences hosted by strangers, and online platforms offering live cooking classes that bridge geographical gaps and create a global dining room. These technological interventions blend customs with contemporary lifestyles, offering new ways to cultivate meaningful connections with food and community in the digital age.

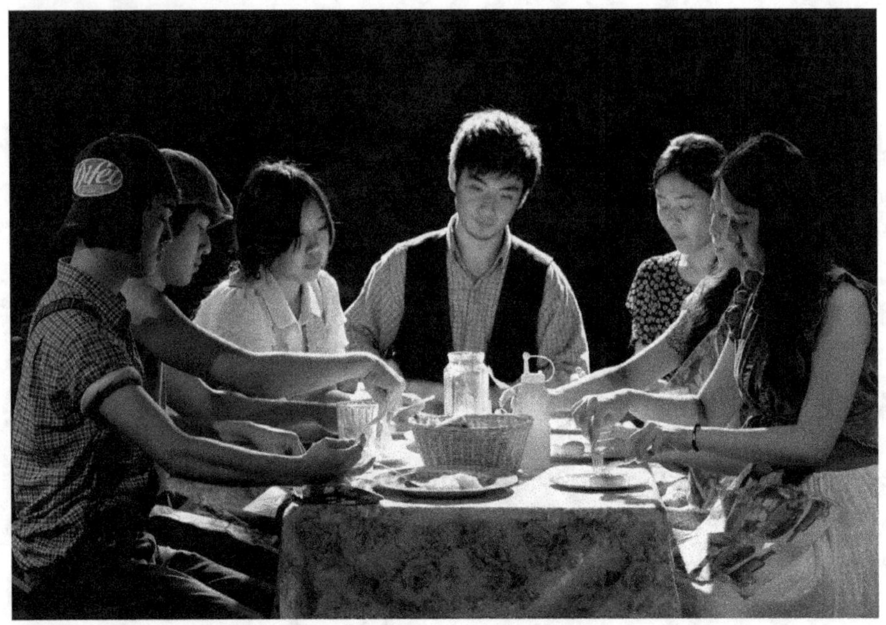

The Role Of Ai In Enhancing Food Rituals

Artificial Intelligence is revolutionizing how we approach nutrition by offering personalized meal plans tailored to individual health data, seasonal ingredients, and mood. By analyzing vast amounts of data, AI systems can suggest recipes that align with users' health goals, dietary restrictions, and flavor preferences, reintroducing the ritual of personalizing meals for health and well-being. This personalized approach makes meal preparation a personal ritual and empowers individuals to make informed, health-conscious decisions about their food choices.

AI also transforms how we perceive and appreciate food by tracing its origins and crafting stories around food items. By providing detailed information about a food's origin, the farmers who grow it, and the landscape it comes from, AI adds depth to the eating experience and fosters a greater appreciation for the hands and lands behind our meals. This integration of storytelling into daily eating rituals enhances our connection with food, making each meal a journey of discovery and appreciation.

AI technologies are being applied to cultivate crop varieties under precisely controlled conditions in vertical farming systems. These farms effectively resurrect ancient seeds with technology by leveraging AI-driven systems to optimize water use, nutrient delivery, and light exposure. This approach produces foods with superior nutritional profiles and flavors and serves as a model for combining historical agricultural wisdom with cutting-edge technology to achieve sustainability and high yield. Through AI-enhanced vertical farming, historic crop varieties are given new life, contributing to a more diverse and resilient food system.

Challenges in Modernizing Rituals

Adopting food rituals into contemporary practices offers opportunities for innovation and adaptation; it also presents challenges that must be carefully navigated. Modernizing food rituals requires a thoughtful and inclusive approach, from the risk of cultural appropriation to the commercialization of traditional practices and the balance between technology use and genuine connections. In this section, we explore the potential challenges and offer strategies for responsibly navigating them to ensure that new rituals are respectful, meaningful, and inclusive.

Cultural Appropriation and Commercialization

Appropriating cultural elements without understanding or respecting their origins can dilute their meaning and exploit them for profit. To address this challenge, it is essential to involve communities in the adaptation process and respect the origins and integrity of traditional practices. This may involve consulting with cultural experts, engaging in dialogue with community members, and ensuring that any adaptations are made with sensitivity and reverence for the cultural heritage being drawn upon.

Balancing Technology and Genuine Connections

Another challenge in modernizing food rituals is striking the right balance between incorporating technology and maintaining genuine connections. While technology offers opportunities for innovation and efficiency, there is a risk of sacrificing meaningful interactions and human connections in favor of convenience and automation. It is crucial to approach technology integration into food rituals thoughtfully, ensuring that it enhances rather than detracts from the authenticity and intimacy of the experience. This may involve using technology to facilitate connections across distances while preserving the human touch and personal engagement central to food rituals.

Addressing Digital Exclusion

Integrating technology in food rituals also presents challenges related to digital exclusion, where only some have equal access to the necessary technologies. This disparity can exacerbate existing inequalities and marginalize specific communities, limiting their participation in adapted present-day food rituals. Addressing this challenge requires policies ensuring more comprehensive access to technology and practical education on using these technologies. Additionally, efforts should be made to develop inclusive platforms and tools that accommodate diverse needs and preferences, ensuring that no one is left behind in the modernization process.

Conclusion

Adapting food rituals for contemporary practices offers exciting possibilities for innovation but also comes with its share of challenges. By addressing issues such as cultural appropriation, commercialization, the balance between technology and genuine connections, and digital exclusion, we can ensure that new rituals are respectful, meaningful, and inclusive. By taking a thoughtful and inclusive approach to modernization, we can preserve the integrity of traditional practices while embracing the opportunities technology offers to enhance today's and tomorrow's food rituals.

CHAPTER 9: NAVIGATING THE INFORMATION WILDERNESS

Introduction: The Digital Dilemma

In today's digital age, we find ourselves immersed in unprecedented information, particularly with respect to food and health. With the rapid growth of digital platforms and the proliferation of user-generated content, the modern digital landscape is teeming with data, presenting opportunities and challenges for consumers seeking to make informed decisions about their diets and lifestyles. However, a significant challenge lies amidst this wealth of information: distinguishing credible information from marketing ploys and misinformation.

According to IBM research, the modern digital landscape is characterized by a deluge of information, with an estimated 90% of the world's data generated in the last 2 years alone (esteramorperez, 2020). This information explosion encompasses various health, nutrition, and sustainability content, ranging from expert opinions and scientific studies to personal anecdotes and marketing messages. While this wealth of information has the potential to empower consumers, it also presents significant challenges in discerning what is credible and trustworthy amidst the noise.

At the heart of this challenge is "digital noise," where misleading advertisements, biased reports, and outright false claims often obscure genuine, helpful information. Studies from the Journal of Marketing have highlighted the impact of constant digital advertising on consumer trust and decision-making, revealing how exposure to persuasive messaging can shape perceptions and influence behavior (Dwivedi et al., 2021). This phenomenon is particularly pronounced when considering food-related health topics, as consumers are bombarded with conflicting messages and exaggerated claims from various sources.

The Role Of Technology In Sifting Truth From Fiction

Technology emerges as a crucial ally in the quest for reliable information amidst the digital deluge, aiding consumers and researchers in sifting truth from fiction. Mainly, advancements in Artificial Intelligence offer promising solutions by enabling the identification of reliable sources and the detection of misinformation.

AI-powered algorithms, utilizing natural language processing and machine learning techniques, are at the forefront of this effort. These algorithms can analyze patterns in data to flag unreliable content and identify biased studies, providing users with tools to navigate the complex landscape of information with greater confidence.

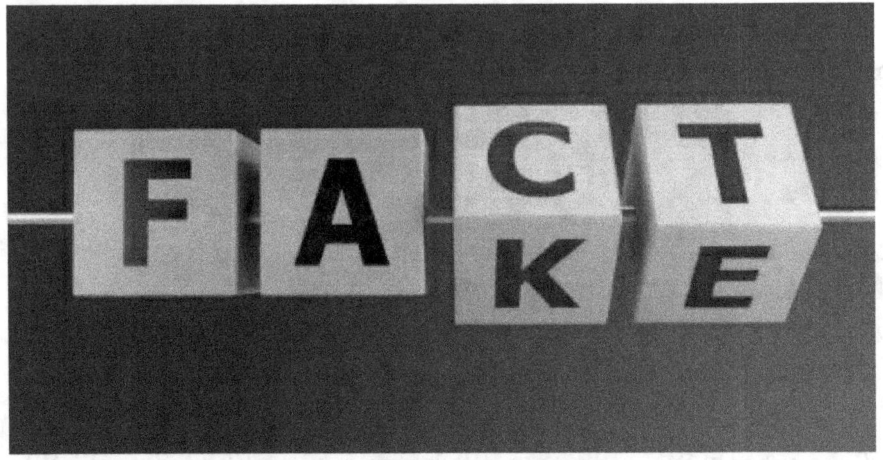

One notable example of utilizing AI in this capacity is HealthFeedback.org, a platform that harnesses expert consensus to evaluate the credibility of viral health claims. By leveraging the collective expertise of qualified professionals, HealthFeedback.org offers consumers a reliable resource for verifying the accuracy of health-related information circulating online.

Furthermore, platforms and apps equipped with AI-driven fact-checking capabilities empower users to make more informed decisions about the credibility of news-related content. For instance, Google's Fact Check Tools enable users to assess the reliability of news articles by pointing to sources that have fact-checked the information. By providing transparent insights into the integrity of online content, these tools help users navigate the digital landscape with discernment and critical thinking.

Incorporating these technological advancements into our information-seeking behaviors enhances our ability to discern truth from fiction. It reinforces the importance of critical thinking and evidence-based decision-making in the digital age. As we harness the power of technology to combat misinformation and promote factual accuracy, we move closer to a more informed and empowered society.

Critical Thinking And Digital Literacy

Critical thinking is a compass in the vast sea of online information, guiding us toward truth and accuracy amidst the noise. At its core, critical thinking involves the ability to analyze, evaluate, and synthesize information in a logical and objective manner. It prompts us to ask probing questions, challenge assumptions, and consider alternative viewpoints before forming conclusions. In the digital realm, where misinformation proliferates unchecked, critical thinking protects against deception and manipulation.

Strategies for Assessing Source Credibility

One of the fundamental pillars of digital literacy is the ability to assess the credibility of online sources. In an age where anyone can easily publish content, distinguishing reliable sources from dubious ones is paramount. To navigate this challenge, individuals can employ various strategies, such as cross-referencing information across multiple sources, scrutinizing the credentials and expertise of authors, and evaluating the reputation of publication platforms. By adopting a vigilant and discerning approach to information consumption, individuals can avoid falling prey to misinformation and propaganda.

Educational Initiatives and Resources: Empowering individuals with the skills necessary to navigate the digital landscape effectively requires concerted efforts from educators, policymakers, and society at large. Educational initiatives and resources play a pivotal role in this regard, providing individuals with the tools and knowledge needed to become savvy consumers and creators of digital content. Organizations like the Stanford History Education Group and projects like the Digital Literacy Project offer valuable resources, including guidelines, curriculum materials, and interactive tools designed to enhance digital literacy skills. By integrating these resources into educational curricula and promoting widespread access, we can foster a generation of digitally literate citizens equipped to thrive in the digital age.

Consumer Empowerment Through Knowledge

Access to accurate and transparent information is pivotal in empowering consumers to make informed choices that support their health goals and ethical values. In today's digital age, where information is readily available, consumers have unprecedented access to data about the products they purchase, from nutritional content to sourcing practices.

Informed consumer choices significantly impact food markets and industries, driving demand for products that prioritize responsible production methods. The rise in consumer awareness about environmental sustainability and animal welfare has increased demand for organically sourced products. This shift in consumer preferences has reshaped the food industry landscape and spurred innovation and investment in more principled practices.

Moreover, access to accurate information can lead to more responsible consumer behaviors, as evidenced by research by the University of Pennsylvania. The study found that transparency in food sourcing builds consumer trust and increases the likelihood of purchasing decisions aligned with personal and environmental health values (Karpyn et al., 2020). When consumers have access to information about where their food comes from and how it is produced, they are better equipped to make choices that support responsible practices and promote overall well-being.

Consumer demand is crucial in influencing food industry practices, prompting companies to respond to informed preferences by offering products that meet higher quality standards and safety. For example, the shift toward non-GMO and organic products reflects a growing awareness among consumers about the potential health and environmental impacts of conventional farming practices. As consumers prioritize transparency and ethical sourcing, they wield significant influence in shaping the future of the food industry and driving positive change toward a more eco-friendly food system.

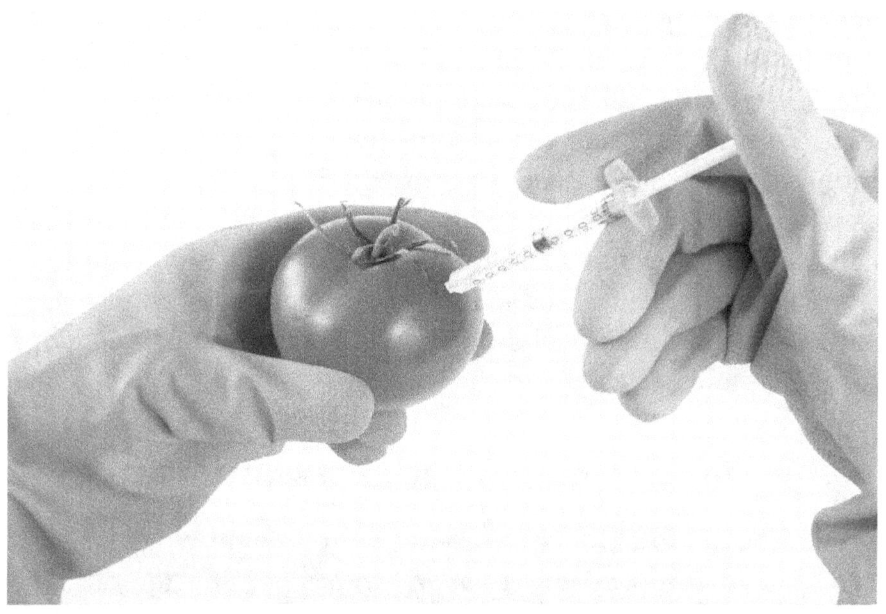

Collaborative Efforts In Information Sharing

Collaborations between academia, industry, and community organizations are crucial in disseminating accurate information about food and nutrition. Successful partnerships have led to impactful public health campaigns and educational programs, highlighting the importance of collective efforts in promoting healthy eating habits and addressing misinformation.

International cooperation is essential in setting standards for food information transparency and regulation. Collaborative initiatives, such as partnerships between the World Health Organization and social media platforms, aim to combat misinformation and ensure users have access to credible sources. Additionally, efforts like the Codex Alimentarius, developed by the Food and Agriculture Organization and World Health

Organization, set internationally recognized food safety and quality standards, facilitating effective information exchange across borders.

Innovative technologies, such as AI-driven systems, are revolutionizing global food safety efforts by monitoring contamination in real time and predicting potential outbreaks. These systems integrate data from diverse sources worldwide, demonstrating the power of international cooperation in proactive health management and disease prevention. Through collaborative initiatives and technology, we are enhancing food safety and setting new standards for global health and well-being, reflecting the historical exchange of food practices and knowledge on a global scale.

Conclusion: Charting A Path Forward

Effective tools and skills are imperative for navigating the food and nutrition complex information landscape. Throughout this chapter, we have explored the importance of critical thinking, digital literacy, and collaboration in discerning truth from fiction amidst the digital noise.

As we conclude, it is evident that a collective effort is needed to cultivate a more informed society where technology and education work hand in hand to empower individuals to make informed choices about their diets and lifestyles. Robust digital literacy and technology tools are essential in cutting through the noise and fostering a healthier, more sustainable relationship with food.

Moving forward, there is a critical need for a multidisciplinary approach combining technology, education, and policy to ensure consumers can access and utilize high-quality information effectively. We can collectively navigate toward a more informed and empowered society by advocating for ongoing global dialogue and policy-making that addresses the digital divide and promotes universal access to reliable information as a fundamental human right. Together, let us embark on this journey toward a future where knowledge is accessible to all and informed choices pave the way for healthier, more sustainable lifestyles.

CHAPTER 10: RECONNECTING THROUGH RITUALS

Introduction: Rediscovering Ancient Pathways

In our journey through "Foraged & Fetched: The Evolutionary Eater's Guide," we've explored the intricate evolution of dietary practices and the profound impact of technology on our food systems. As we delve into Chapter 10, "Reconnecting Through Rituals," we aim to bridge the gap between ancient wisdom and innovation, exploring how technology can breathe new life into age-old food rituals.

Understanding The Power Of Rituals In Human History

Throughout history, rituals have been pillars of human culture, shaping our identities and fostering community bonds. From feasts celebrating seasonal harvests to elaborate ceremonies marking life milestones, rituals around food have played a central role in human societies worldwide. These practices nourished and served as avenues for social cohesion and cultural expression.

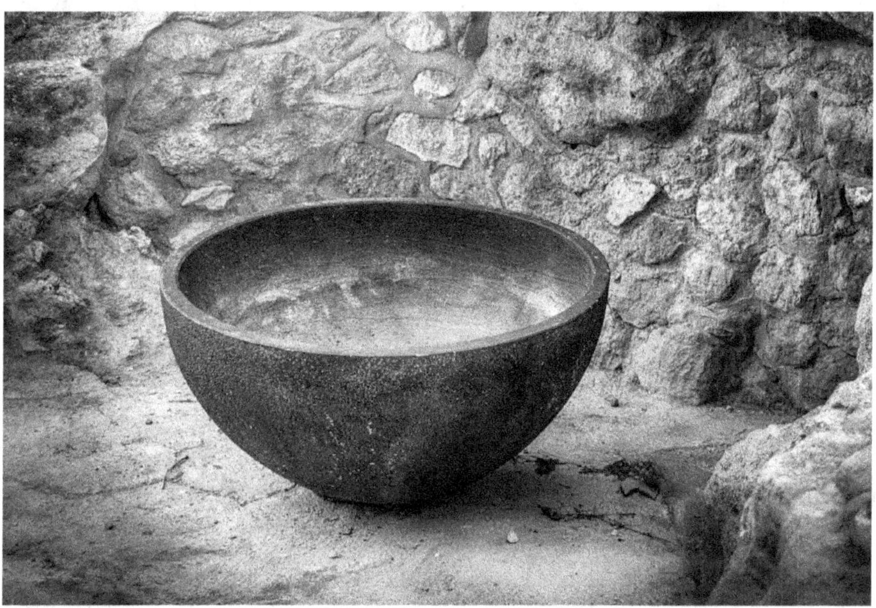

Consider the historical civilizations of Mesopotamia, where the New Year's feast ritual was a cornerstone of societal cohesion and religious devotion. In Mesopotamian culture, the Akitu festival began the agricultural year with a grand feast with offerings to the gods, communal banquets, and symbolic rituals representing life's cyclical nature and the earth's renewal. This annual celebration not only served to honor the gods and ensure the fertility of the land but also fostered a sense of unity and solidarity among the people, strengthening social bonds and reinforcing shared cultural values.

Similarly, in ancient Egypt, the ritual of the annual flooding of the Nile was accompanied by elaborate feasts and ceremonies, commemorating the divine forces responsible for the inundation and celebrating the abundance it brought to the land. These feasts, held in temples and palaces across the kingdom, sustain the populace's physical bodies and nourish their souls, fostering a deep connection to the natural world and the divine forces that governed it.

Moving forward in history, we encounter the elaborate food rituals of the medieval European court, where feasting was elevated to an art form and a means of asserting power and prestige. In the courts of kings and nobles, lavish banquets were orchestrated with meticulous attention to detail, showcasing the wealth and sophistication of the ruling elite. These feasts, characterized by extravagant displays of food and drink, served not only to entertain and delight but also to reinforce social hierarchies and political alliances, cementing the bonds of loyalty and allegiance among the aristocracy.

The Disconnection: Modern Challenges And Loss Of Traditions

However, industrialization and digitalization have gradually eroded these time-honored food rituals. In our fast-paced, convenience-driven world, communal meals have been replaced by solitary fast food consumption, contributing to social isolation and disconnection from our food sources. This loss of tradition not only impacts our well-being but also threatens the resilience of our communities and the sustainability of our food systems.

Technology As A Catalyst For Reconnection

Yet, amidst these challenges, technology is a powerful catalyst for rekindling our connection to food rituals. Platforms like "EatWith" and virtual reality applications enable us to recreate communal dining experiences and immerse ourselves in the culinary traditions of our ancestors. By leveraging advanced tools, we can revive practices in ways that resonate with contemporary lifestyles, fostering a sense of continuity and cultural pride.

Case Studies: Rituals In Action

The Slow Food Movement is a shining example of how technology can amplify the revival of traditional food practices globally. Slow Food promotes local and sustainable food systems through digital platforms and social media, preserving culinary diversity and celebrating indigenous food cultures. Similarly, online platforms offering virtual cooking classes empower individuals to learn and share culinary techniques, ensuring these traditions endure in the digital age.

Founded in Italy in 1986, Slow Food emerged as a response to the encroaching homogenization of global diets and the loss of traditional culinary practices. Today, it has evolved into a global grassroots organization dedicated to promoting locally responsible food systems, preserving culinary diversity, and celebrating indigenous food cultures.

At the heart of the Slow Food Movement lies a deep appreciation for the rituals and traditions that have sustained communities for generations. Slow Food amplifies its message to a global audience through its digital platforms and social media channels. From virtual farmers' markets to online cooking tutorials, these digital initiatives enable individuals to connect with local producers, discover traditional recipes, and participate in the revival of food rituals.

One notable example of Slow Food's digital innovation is the "Ark of Taste," an online catalog documenting and celebrating endangered food products worldwide. By raising awareness of these culinary treasures, Slow Food aims to protect and preserve traditional foodways, ensuring that future generations can continue to savor their heritage flavors.

Online Cooking Classes: Empowering Culinary Exploration

In an era dominated by convenience foods and fast-casual dining, home cooking is experiencing a resurgence, thanks partly to the proliferation of online cooking classes. Platforms like MasterClass, Udemy, and YouTube offer a wealth of resources for aspiring chefs and home cooks, providing step-by-step tutorials on everything from basic knife skills to complex pastry techniques. There are even courses tailored for every age group, including kids, like Raddish Kids Cooking Club and Kidstir.

But beyond mere instruction, online cooking classes serve as a gateway to the world of culinary traditions, allowing individuals to explore the rich tapestry of global cuisine from the comfort of their kitchens. Whether mastering the art of sushi-making or learning the secrets of French patisserie, these virtual culinary adventures enable participants to connect with the cultural heritage and ancestral wisdom embedded in traditional food rituals.

By democratizing access to culinary knowledge and expertise, online cooking classes empower individuals to reclaim control over their diets and rediscover the joy of cooking. Whether preserving family recipes passed down through generations or experimenting with new flavors and techniques, participants in these digital culinary journeys are forging deeper connections to their food and heritage.

Building New Rituals: Practical Steps For Individuals And Communities

Practical steps are within reach for those seeking to reconnect with their food heritage. Digital food diaries and seasonal food apps facilitate mindful eating and local consumption, while AI-driven nutrition recommendations offer personalized guidance rooted in timeless dietary wisdom. By embracing these tools, individuals and communities can rediscover the joy of shared meals and the richness of cultural food traditions.

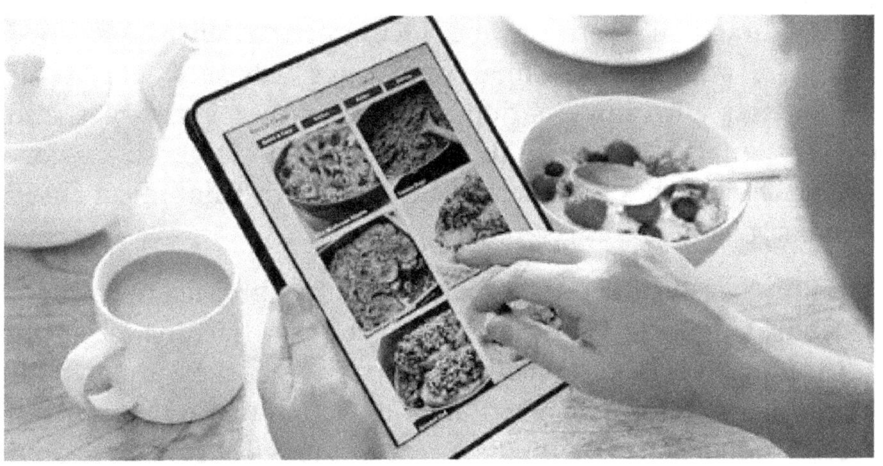

Keeping Digital Food Diaries: A Modern Twist on an Ancient Practice

One practical step toward building new food rituals is adopting digital food diaries. These online tools enable individuals to track their daily food intake, monitor nutritional content, and reflect on their eating habits. While the concept of food diaries may seem novel to some, it hearkens back to traditions of mindful eating and self-reflection.

For example, in Ayurvedic medicine, practitioners often recommend keeping a food journal to understand the effects of different foods on the body and mind. By recording what they eat and how it makes them feel, individuals can gain insight into their unique dietary needs and make informed choices that promote health and well-being.

In the digital age, platforms like MyFitnessPal and Lose It! have taken this concept to the next level, offering users a user-friendly interface and a wealth of features to track their dietary intake and set personalized health goals. By incorporating these tools into their daily routines, individuals can become more aware of their food choices and develop healthier eating habits over time.

Seasonal Food Apps: Embracing the Rhythms of Nature

Another practical step toward reconnecting with our food heritage is adopting seasonal food apps. These digital tools provide users with information on which fruits, vegetables, and other seasonal foods are currently available in their region, allowing them to make informed choices about what to eat based on what's fresh and in season.

In many cultures, eating seasonally is deeply ingrained in culinary traditions. It reflects an understanding of the rhythms of nature and the importance of consuming foods when they are at their peak in terms of flavor, nutrition, and availability. By embracing seasonal food apps, individuals can reconnect with aged wisdom and rediscover the joy of eating locally grown and harvested foods at their freshest.

One example of a seasonal food app is Harvest, which provides users with real-time information on the availability of seasonal produce in their area. This app allows individuals to plan their meals around what's in season, supporting local farmers and reducing their carbon footprint.

The Future Of Food Rituals

Looking ahead, the future of food rituals holds boundless possibilities. As AI technology evolves, personalized nutrition recommendations will become increasingly tailored to individual needs, seamlessly blending ancient wisdom with modern science. Moreover, global collaborations and initiatives, such as the Codex Alimentarius, will set international standards for food transparency and quality, ensuring that traditional food practices remain accessible and respected worldwide.

AI-Driven Nutrition Recommendations:
Personalized Guidance Rooted in Tradition

In addition to digital food diaries and seasonal food apps, another practical step toward building new food rituals is adopting AI-driven nutrition recommendations. These cutting-edge tools use advanced algorithms to analyze individuals' dietary habits, health goals, and nutritional needs, providing personalized guidance rooted in dietary wisdom.

For example, apps like Nutrino and Fooducate leverage AI technology to offer users personalized meal plans and nutritional advice based on their unique health profiles. By considering age, gender, activity level, and dietary preferences, these apps can recommend foods that align with individuals' health goals and cultural preferences.

In addition to AI-driven personalized nutrition, the future of food rituals will be shaped by global collaborations and initiatives to set international standards for food transparency and quality. Organizations like the Codex Alimentarius, established by the Food and Agriculture Organization and the World Health Organization, will play a pivotal role in this endeavor, ensuring that traditional food practices remain accessible and respected worldwide.

Conclusion: Embracing The Past To Inform The Future

In conclusion, Chapter 10 underscores the importance of reconnecting with our dietary past to inform a healthier, more sustainable future. By integrating rituals with modern technology, we can forge deeper connections with our food, communities, and cultural heritage. As we embrace this journey of rediscovery, let us harness the power of technology to honor our ancestors, nourish our bodies, and cultivate a world where food rituals enrich our lives for generations to come.

CONCLUSION

*Harmonizing Our Ancestral
Needs With Technology*

As we conclude our exploration in "Foraged & Fetched: The Evolutionary Eater's Guide," we reflect on a journey that has traversed the expansive landscapes of human history, from our primal origins to the present-day technological era. Each chapter has progressively uncovered the deep connections between our biological evolution and diets, illuminating how these relationships have shaped our physical forms, societies, and environments.

Throughout this book, we've seen how ancient dietary practices, honed over millennia, provided our ancestors with the nutrients necessary for robust health and the development of complex societies. However, as we ventured into the modern age, the advent of industrial agriculture and mass food production began to distort these time-honored connections. The result has been a profound disruption in our diets and the ecological balance that once dictated human and non-human life rhythms.

Yet, this narrative does not end with a lament for what has been lost. Instead, it extends a hopeful vision for the future, where technology is a powerful tool to restore and even enhance our ancestral dietary practices. We've discussed innovative tools, from AI in nutritional planning to blockchain in food traceability, that can help us reclaim the authenticity of our diets, offering promising solutions.

The benefits of aligning our advanced capabilities with ecological and biological wisdom are not just theoretical but tangible and impactful. By doing so, we can forge food systems that are not only efficient but also ethical and sustainable. This approach doesn't just feed the world; it nourishes it, respecting the complex web of life that sustains us all.

In this spirit, we emphasize each reader's crucial role in our future narrative. Inspired by this book's insights, your personal and community actions, whether supporting local agriculture, engaging in foraging apps, or advocating for sustainable food policies, contribute to a larger movement toward dietary enlightenment and ecological stewardship.

Finally, as we look to the future, we envision a world enriched by a synergy between technological prowess and primal dietary wisdom. This is not merely a return to the past but a progression toward a future where our technologies support reconnection with our natural dietary roots, enhancing our health and planet.

In embracing this balanced approach, we rekindle our primal connections to our food, the earth, and each other, forging a path that respects our heritage while innovatively addressing contemporary challenges. Though complex, this journey promises a harmonious future where the fusion of technology and tradition breathes new life into our global foodscapes.

References

Abrams, Z. (2021, March 1). *Controlling the spread of misinformation.* American Psychological Association. https://www.apa.org/monitor/2021/03/controlling-misinformation

Bensinger, G. (2023, February 21). Focus: ChatGPT launches boom in AI-written e-books on Amazon. *Reuters.* https://www.reuters.com/technology/chatgpt-launches-boom-ai-written-e-books-amazon-2023-02-21/

Bohn, R. E., & Short, J. E. (2010, January). *HMI? How much information?* Global Information Industry Center. https://group47.com/HMI_2009_ConsumerReport_Dec9_2009.pdf

Bristol, N. (2020, June 9). *The U.S. Government and Antimicrobial Resistance.* CSIS. https://www.csis.org/analysis/us-government-and-antimicrobial-resistance

Brown, S. (2020, October 5). *MIT Sloan research about social media, misinformation, and elections.* MIT Sloan; MIT Sloan School of Management. https://mitsloan.mit.edu/ideas-made-to-matter/mit-sloan-research-about-social-media-misinformation-and-elections

Chen, J. C., Aldenderfer, M., Eerkens, J. W., Langlie, B. S., Carlos Viviano Llave, Watson, J. T., & Haas, R. (2024). Stable isotope chemistry reveals plant-dominant diet among early foragers on the Andean Altiplano, 9.0–6.5 cal. ka. *PLOS ONE, 19*(1), e0296420–e0296420. https://doi.org/10.1371/journal.pone.0296420

Conroy, G. (2023, June 22). *Hunter-gatherer lifestyle fosters thriving gut microbiome.* Nature. https://doi.org/10.1038/d41586-023-02065-y

Cuthbertson, A. (2023, February 22). *Hundreds*

of AI-written books flood Amazon. *The Independent.* https://www.independent.co.uk/tech/ai-author-books-amazon-chatgpt-b2287111.html

Dadgostar, P. (2019). Antimicrobial resistance: Implications and costs. *Infection and Drug Resistance, 12*(12), 3903–3910. https://doi.org/10.2147/idr.s234610

Diamond, H., & Diamond, M. (2010). *Fit for Life.* Wellness Central.

Diamond, J. (2008). *Guns, Germs, and Steel the Fates of Human Societies.* Paw Prints.

Dwivedi, Y. K., Ismagilova, E., Hughes, D. L., Carlson, J., Filieri, R., Jacobson, J., Jain, V., Karjaluoto, H., Kefi, H., Krishen, A. S., Kumar, V., Rahman, M. M., Raman, R., Rauschnabel, P. A., Rowley, J., Salo, J., Tran, G. A., & Wang, Y. (2021, August). Setting the future of digital and social media marketing research: Perspectives and research propositions. *International Journal of Information Management, 59*(1), 1–37. https://doi.org/10.1016/j.ijinfomgt.2020.102168

esteramorperez. (2020, May 28). *How to manage complexity and realize the value of big data.* IBM Blog. https://www.ibm.com/blog/how-to-manage-complexity-and-realize-the-value-of-big-data/

Fragiadakis, G. K., Smits, S. A., Sonnenburg, E. D., William Van Treuren, Reid, G., Knight, R., Alphaxard Manjurano, Changalucha, J., Maria Gloria Dominguez-Bello, Leach, J., & Sonnenburg, J. L. (2018). Links between environment, diet, and the hunter-gatherer microbiome. *BioRxiv (Cold Spring Harbor Laboratory).* https://pubmed.ncbi.nlm.nih.gov/30118385/

GOV.UK. (2018). *Data Protection Act 2018.* The National Archives | legislation.gov.uk. https://www.legislation.gov.uk/ukpga/2018/12/contents/enacted

Gunagi, P. R., Karikatti, S. S., & Halki, S. B. (2019). Assessment of knowledge of risk factors and prevention of obesity among school children: A cross-sectional study. *International Journal of Community Medicine and Public Health, 7*(1), 111. https://doi.org/10.18203/2394-6040.ijcmph20195838

Hitchcock, R., & Babchuk, W. (2007). Kalahari San foraging, land use, and territoriality: Implications for the future. *Before Farming, 2007*(3), 1–14. https://doi.org/10.3828/bfarm.2007.3.3

Jantan, I., Bukhari, S. N. A., Mohamed, M. A. S., Wai, L. K., & Mesaik, M. A. (2015, June 3). *The evolving role of natural products from the tropical rainforests as a replenishable source of new drug leads.* In Drug Discovery and Development - From Molecules to Medicine. https://www.intechopen.com/chapters/47844

Karpyn, A., McCallops, K., Wolgast, H., & Glanz, K. (2020, October 16). Improving consumption and purchases of healthier foods in retail environments: A systematic review. *Int. J. Environ. Res. Public Health, 17*(20), 7524. https://doi.org/10.3390/ijerph17207524

Klurfeld, D. M., Foreyt, J., Angelopoulos, T. J., & Rippe, J. M. (2012). Lack of evidence for high fructose corn syrup as the cause of the obesity epidemic. *International Journal of Obesity, 37*(6), 771–773. https://doi.org/10.1038/ijo.2012.157

Lee, R. B. (1979). *The !Kung San: Men and women work in a foraging society.* Cambridge University Press.

Lindeberg, S., Eliasson, M., Lindahl, B., & Ahrén, B. (1999). Low serum insulin in traditional pacific islanders—The Kitava study. *Metabolism, 48*(10), 1216. https://www.academia.edu/9412333/Low_serum_insulin_in_traditional_pacific_islanders_The_Kitava_study

Methadone for opioid addiction: Benefits and risks - Haven Detox

Little Rock. (2023, December 1). The Haven Detox. https://arkansasrecovery.com/methadone-treatment/methadone-for-opioid-addiction-benefits-and-risks/

Morgenstern, J. D., Rosella, L. C., Costa, A. P., de Souza, R. J., & Anderson, L. N. (2021). Perspective: Big data and machine learning could help advance nutritional epidemiology. *Advances in Nutrition (Bethesda, Md.)*, *12*(3), 621–631. https://doi.org/10.1093/advances/nmaa183

Moubtahij, Z., Jaouen, K., & Jacob, S. (2024, April 29). *More plants on the menu of ancient hunter-gatherers.* Max-Planck-Gesellschaft. https://www.mpg.de/21865602/more-plants-on-the-menu-of-ancient-hunters-gatherers

Muhammed, S. T., & Mathew, S. K. (2022). The disaster of misinformation: A review of research in social media. *International Journal of Data Science and Analytics*, *13*(4), 271–285. https://www.ncbi.nlm.nih.gov/pmc/articles/PMC8853081/

O'Neill, J. (2016). Tackling drug-resistant infections globally: Final report and recommendations. *Archives of Pharmacy Practice*, *7*(3), 110. https://doi.org/10.4103/2045-080x.186181

Palosky, C. (2021, November 8). *COVID-19 misinformation is ubiquitous: 78% of the public believes or is unsure about at least one false statement, and nearly a third believe at least four of eight false statements tested.* KFF. https://www.kff.org/coronavirus-covid-19/press-release/covid-19-misinformation-is-ubiquitous-78-of-the-public-believes-or-is-unsure-about-at-least-one-false-statement-and-nearly-at-third-believe-at-least-four-of-eight-false-statements-tested/

Roetzel, P. G. (2018). Information overload in the information age: A literature review from business administration, business psychology, and related disciplines with a bibliometric approach and framework development. *Business Research*,

12(2). https://doi.org/10.1007/s40685-018-0069-z

Temple, N. J. (2022). The origins of the obesity epidemic in the USA–Lessons for Today. *Nutrients*, 14(20), 4253. National Library of Medicine. https://doi.org/10.3390/nu14204253

Skorbiansky, S. R., Carlson, A., & Spalding, A. (2023, November 14). *USDA ERS - Rising consumer demand reshapes landscape for U.S. organic farmers.* USDA ERS. https://www.ers.usda.gov/amber-waves/2023/november/rising-consumer-demand-reshapes-landscape-for-u-s-organic-farmers/

Villegas, R., Yang, G., Gao, Y.-T. ., Cai, H., Li, H., Zheng, W., & Shu, X. O. (2010). Dietary patterns are associated with lower incidence of type 2 diabetes in middle-aged women: The Shanghai Women's Health Study. *International Journal of Epidemiology, 39*(3), 889–899. https://doi.org/10.1093/ije/dyq008

Wendorf, M. (2019, March 29). *High fructose corn syrup and the obesity epidemic.* Interesting Engineering. https://interestingengineering.com/health/high-fructose-corn-syrup-and-the-obesity-epidemic

Yellen, J. E. (1990). The transformation of the Kalahari !Kung. *Scientific American, 262*(4), 96–105. https://www.jstor.org/stable/24996723

Images

andrelyra. (2014, March 24). *Technology, informatics, computers image.* Pixabay. https://pixabay.com/photos/technology-informatics-computers-298256

andyballard. (2016, January 27). *Samphire, foraging, nature image.* Pixabay. https://pixabay.com/photos/samphire-foraging-nature-1164952

Angeleses. (2018, July 11). *Vessel, bowl, ceramics image*. Pixabay. https://pixabay.com/photos/vessel-bowl-ceramics-antiquity-3530090

artursfoto. (2016, October 16). *Modified, tomato, genetically image*. Pixabay. https://pixabay.com/photos/modified-tomato-genetically-food-1744952

Blogcube. (2021, November 21). *Oil, medicinal, healthy image*. Pixabay. https://pixabay.com/photos/oil-medicinal-healthy-herbs-plant-6810988

brenkee. (2016, March 26). *Fermented, cucumber, glass image*. Pixabay. https://pixabay.com/photos/fermented-cucumber-glass-food-1280682

Character, theater stage, monologue image. (2014, August28). Pixabay. https://pixabay.com/photos/character-theater-stage-monologue-430564

danramirez. (2016, June23). *Coffee grains, mature, farming image*. Pixabay. https://pixabay.com/photos/coffee-grains-mature-farming-plant-1474601

Eoneren. (2018, July 25). *Fact or fake concept with wooden cubes stock photo*. Pixabay. https://www.istockphoto.com/photo/fact-or-fake-concept-with-wooden-cubes-gm1007097736-271758296

geralt. (2018, July 13). *Network, Earth, blockchain image*. Pixabay. https://pixabay.com/photos/network-earth-blockchain-globe-3537394

Jackson, B. (2014, October 20). *Sockeye, salmon, Kenai image*. Pixabay. https://pixabay.com/photos/sockeye-salmon-kenai-fish-wild-492258

Just_Super. (2024, January 22). *AI for good*. Pixabay. https://www.istockphoto.com/collaboration/boards/

L1epD0mmG0KxRXQkX_BLng

kaboompics. (2015, May 30). *Basil, cup, nature image*. Pixabay. https://pixabay.com/photos/basil-cup-herbs-green-leaf-leaves-791781

Marijana1. (2018, September 22). *Smoothie, nutrition, detox image*. Pixabay. https://pixabay.com/photos/smoothie-nutrition-detox-juice-3697014

matthiasboeckel. (2019, December 1). *Grilling, salmon, fish image*. Pixabay. https://pixabay.com/photos/grilling-salmon-fish-grill-healthy-4665509

monkeybusinessimages. (2015, September 2). *Person at breakfast looking at recipe app on digital tablet stock photo*. Pixabay. https://www.istockphoto.com/photo/person-at-breakfast-looking-at-recipe-app-on-digital-tablet-gm486507818-73016847

Pexels. (2016, November 18). *Apples, farmer's market, buy image*. Pixabay. https://pixabay.com/photos/apples-farmers-market-buy-buying-1841132

proths. (2019, December 4). *Tea, tea ceremony, tea cup image*. Pixabay. https://pixabay.com/photos/tea-tea-ceremony-tea-cup-china-4674073

Tumisu. (2021, January 26). *Man, face, facial recognition image*. Pixabay. https://pixabay.com/photos/man-face-facial-recognition-5946820/

Yeppo. (2020, September 24). *Berries, nature, raspberry image*. Pixabay. https://pixabay.com/photos/berries-raspberry-strawberry-fruit-5597501

www.ingramcontent.com/pod-product-compliance
Lightning Source LLC
Chambersburg PA
CBHW051817250726
48659CB00005B/1530